Hugh Lasgarn grew up in a small Welsh village and trained at Glasgow Veterinary College. Since graduating, he has lived and worked in the Welsh Border country that he loves and where he met and married his wife. A devoted healer of animals great and small, he believes that the essential ingredient for a vet is not love of animals but respect for them, combined with the incentive to ease suffering and the courage to take life when pain is beyond control.

VET IN GREEN PASTURES

Hugh Lasgarn

Fontana/Collins

First published by Souvenir Press Ltd 1985
First issued in Fontana Paperbacks 1986

Copyright © Souvenir Press 1985

Made and printed in Great Britain by
William Collins Sons & Co. Ltd, Glasgow

To Mother

It is not a love of animals that makes a vet, but rather a respect for them. A respect for their feelings when sick or injured, an awareness of their reactions when frightened.

Add to this the incentive to cure disease and ease suffering and the courage to take a life when pain is beyond control — and you have the essential ingredients.

But where to begin?

For me, it was in a small village in Wales . . .

Hugh Lasgarn
September 1984

One

If, to you, chocolate biscuits are still 'special' and roast chicken still a 'treat'; if, when aeroplanes fly overhead at night, you keep your eyes fixed firmly upon the ground, then you were probably, like me, about seven when the War started. And at that age, becoming a country vet could hardly have been further from my mind.

The austerity that accompanied that conflict was not too great a hardship for the folks of Abergranog, for the community had never indulged in luxuries, due to a combination of hard times and a strong religious doctrine that anything enjoyable was bad for the soul.

It would be hypocritical to deny youngsters of today the pleasures they seem to take for granted, for in Abergranog in those days we had enough. The leavening of wartime restrictions did nothing more than prolong the status quo and keep us slim and eager and very much on our toes for any information as to the whereabouts of 'specials'.

'There's bananas in Powell the Fruit!' I remember the cry well, and that I ran all the way down to the shop . . . but I never saw any.

I did see the lemon that John Pope's father brought back when he came on leave. We raffled it at school for the War Effort. I would have given my right arm to have won it that day.

The whole school was allowed to feel it.

'Just feel it and don't squeeze it,' were the instructions. But some boys — Boxy Potter was one — squeezed it hard.

1

So did I. So it can't have been much cop.

So much for 'treats' and 'specials'. But it was Mr Talfyn Thomas who was responsible for the night flying tactics we were advised to adopt; in fact, he frightened the pants off our butties one day when he told us all about air raids.

Mr Talfyn Thomas was Chief Warden for Abergranog and came to talk to us at school in the Big Hall. He came in his Chapel suit, tie on as well, with the little cutty-back collar, a tin helmet, gas mask, arm band with ARP written on it and a bucket of sand which he placed beside him.

'What does ARP stand for?' he shouted, in the same voice he used in temperance classes, where we had to go to learn about drinking.

'A Runty Pig!' whispered Boxy Potter behind me, and we all laughed, but Talfyn was oblivious to that remark, for he was lost in his zeal to save Abergranog from the Germans.

He told us about the sirens and fire watching and what to do with the sand, and it all sounded most exciting. At last he came to the 'blackout' and the danger of showing lights at night. He narrowed his eyes and lowered his voice to a hiss, as he did when he talked about 'The Devil's Brew'.

'At night, 'ew boys, at night if 'ew'm out an' 'ew hears Jerry overhead, don't look up! Don't look up, for 'ewer eyes do shine like cats' in the dark! An' if 'e sees 'ew...' He threw his arms in the air and shouted: 'IT'S BOOM BOOM! GOODBYE, DAIO!'

I never forgot it.

But there was fun to be had, too, slipping newts into cardboard gasmask boxes, sticking window tape over girls' spectacles or filling inkwells with sand. The summer was fine, with ripe whinberries thick on the Incline, apples to be scrumped and the hedgerows full of blackberries.

To add to all this, I had an unexpected bonus. In fact, it was Mr Talfyn Thomas who was instrumental in one of the major achievements of my boyhood days and, maybe,

2

even beyond.

I was allowed legal access to Little Pant.

Little Pant was the farm at the back of our house. It was made up of three lumpy cow pastures in the shape of an 'L', with a small cow house and barn in the angle.

Five fat and happy cows lived off the uneven sward, tended by Arty Parry, who also delivered milk. The owners were the Misses Prowle, two sisters who were very proper and described by Mother as 'a bit tetchy'.

It was easy to scramble over our back wall and make sorties into the fields. They were of the old-fashioned type, rare today, for they were permanent to a degree. Uneven, lush, tussocky grass with scattered coltsfoot and buttercup, and clutches of thistles growing in odd patches that were occasionally scythed wearily by Arty.

Throughout the pasture lay hidden, like some manurial minefield, cowpats in various stages of crusted maturity, that attracted hordes of buzzing brown flies, multicoloured beetles and small boys' boots.

That was one of the reasons I was forbidden in the fields, the other being that the Misses Prowle didn't like trespassers.

My passport to Little Pant came as a result of 'Air Raid Dispersal', as explained in the Big Hall by Mr Talfyn Thomas. In the event of an air raid during school time, all children living within half a mile would be allowed home. Those living beyond the 'safe distance' would have to go to a friend's house within the limit.

Because I lived over a mile by road, I was allocated a place in Wendel Weekes' house. His father was a bus driver with Western Welsh and bred wire-haired fox terriers. Wendel was a good friend of mine and I welcomed the choice . . . although I would have much preferred to go straight home.

It was Miss Webb, our teacher, who gave me the idea when she was telling us about maps, and how black lines were for rivers and stripes for railways, brown for high ground and green for low.

'"As the crow flies",' she said in her sing-song voice, 'means that if a crow was to fly, say, from school to Abergranog Park, it wouldn't go round the road, it would go straight from here over the farm and into the park. Much quicker it would be, wouldn't it?'

I lived on Bowen's Pitch next to the park and I was on to it like a shot.

I bit my pen handle hard with excitement, waiting for class to end so that I could tell Miss Webb of my scheme.

'"As the crow flies",' I told her confidently, 'I could be home very quickly if I went through Little Pant. Mother would be very pleased if I could, because she gets worried if I'm in school an' there are Germans about.'

She listened to my explanation and said she would have to talk to Mr Talfyn Thomas.

To my surprise and delight, it worked. Subject to certain conditions, I would be allowed to go through Little Pant in order to get home during an air raid.

The conditions were, firstly, that the Misses Prowle should give permission and, secondly, that Miss Webb should come with me on a trial trip to ensure it was all right.

The Misses Prowle agreed, for both Mr Talfyn Thomas and they were big Chapel people and, subject to Miss Webb sanctioning the route, I had made it.

The day she came with me it had been raining and she walked with high, stilty steps to try and keep her shoes dry.

The cows were in the second field, and when we started across I felt her hand grip mine so tightly that my fingers stuck together.

'You're not afraid of cows, Hugh?' she asked, in a shrill voice.

'No, Miss Webb,' I replied, manfully. And neither was I, for I had been across the field many times, illegally of course, and they had taken not the slightest bit of notice.

She quickened her step, forgetting the wet grass as we skirted the grazing bunch.

4

'Have they got names?' she asked, breathing rather fast.

'Yes, Miss Webb. And I know them all.' To have Miss Webb all to myself and to teach her about the cows was making my day.

'The big grey is Old Blod and the little grey is Young Blod,' I explained. 'Because she's her daughter. The red cow looking at us is called Lewis, because she came from Mr Lewis, Ty-Canol. The little brown one is very special because she is pedigree. Her name is Cystrema Golden Platter, but we call her Cis.'

'And the big black one?' she asked, nervously.

I savoured the moment. It had had to come and I wondered whether she would react as the Misses Prowle had done when they called one day and Mother proudly asked me to name the cows.

'The black one,' I said, looking up into her face, 'is called Old Thundertits!'

Miss Webb did react, though not quite as obviously as the Misses Prowle. I don't need to explain, of course, that Arty had let the name slip and that she was really called Blackie.

I suppose it was a wicked thing to long for an air raid, but I did, and I had to wait three weeks for the siren to blow in school time.

It came one Wednesday, just after dinner time, and, with instructions to go speedily home, class was abandoned. I set off down the road for the gate to Little Pant. Once inside the first field I slackened pace and scuffed delightedly through the long grass.

I was halfway across the second field, which I thought was empty, when I saw her, Old Thundertits, lying on her side, all by herself.

She seemed such an odd shape, her stomach blown up like a drum, and she was grunting great squirts of steam from her nose. I stood and watched for some minutes before I plucked up courage to draw closer.

Her one horn was covered in fresh soil where it had been

digging in the ground and her eyes were stary and unblinking. It was only when I was very close that I noticed the lump beneath her tail. It was large and balloon-like and shimmered in the afternoon sun.

Every time she grunted it grew bigger and, when it suddenly moved, I held my breath.

I stood transfixed as the lump elongated, wriggled and writhed behind the old cow. Suddenly I was conscious of a droning in the air above, but I couldn't take my eyes off the swelling behind the straining legs. Old Thundertits was gasping, then the shape grew suddenly much bigger and the droning sound louder. For a fleeting second a great shadow covered us both, then there was a 'pop', the balloon burst and amid a rush of brown water I saw two small feet and a head appear. It was a baby calf.

Although I'd never seen anything like it in my life before, I didn't feel frightened or ill — just mesmerised. Then the feet moved up and down as if waving at me and the mouth partly opened to give out a watery bawling sound. Still moving its feet, it bawled again, then pushed out a short pink tongue that curled up to its nose.

I was in no doubt that the little creature was asking for help, so I squatted down and took hold of one of the legs with both hands.

I shall never, ever forget the sensation. Warm and tacky it was, but it was the wonderful feeling of life, even though it was just a leg, that thrilled the whole of my tingling body.

The leg plucked back a shade, but I didn't let go. Then it came forward about six inches; I re-adjusted my squat and pulled gently, and the little creature came forward even more. Both legs were now clear to the shoulders and the head was quite free. Suddenly, Old Thundertits gave one mighty heave and the calf shot halfway out, accompanied by a great flood that ran all around my boots. I stood up a little, and as I did there was another heave and out it came — all of it — wet and still bawling and its big brown eyes blinking in the light.

I stayed and watched the old lady get up and lick her newborn. It was unbelievable how quickly it tried to stand. I made a move to help but Old Thundertits moaned at me, so I left it alone.

It was only when All-Clear sounded that I remembered about the air raid and, running through the cow pats, I sped home to tell Mother.

It was all the talk of Abergranog the following day. Quite a lot of folk had seen the stray Heinkel He III, with the black cross and swastika on its tail, sail up the valley.

'I saw the German pilot,' said Boxy Potter. 'Clear as anything. Come right over our garden, just as I got home.'

The rest of the class listened in awe as Boxy described the sight. Even Miss Webb let him have full rein, and he made the most of it.

'You must have seen it!' He looked over to my desk with a superior sneer on his spotty face. 'It come right over Little Pant as 'ew was goin' home.'

The eyes of Class Two fell upon me.

'Did 'ew see it?' asked Wendel.

'No. I didn't,' I replied.

'Hidin' 'ewer eyes, was 'ew?' Boxy chimed in sarcastically.

The whole class laughed and waited for my reaction.

'I was watching a calf bein' born,' I said nonchalantly.

There were gasps of surprise and admiration. Boxy sat down and I knew I had stolen his glory.

'Was this at Little Pant, Hugh?' Miss Webb took up the management of the class again.

'Yes, Miss.'

'Which cow was the mother?'

'Old ... Blackie, Miss.' Miss Webb gave a short gasp, then smiled.

'Now that was interesting. Come up to the front and tell us all about it.'

So up to the front I went and told them.

I described the experience with such graphic detail that,

when I came to the part where all the skin and brown jelly came oozing out, Boxy Potter had to leave the room.

That pleased me no end.

When I had finished I went back to my seat feeling pretty good.

*   *   *

If that experience did anything to guide me into the veterinary profession I certainly wasn't aware of it at the time. But no doubt, subconsciously, it started me on a trail that otherwise I might never have known.

The valley environment, while not conducive to veterinary practice, was not completely devoid of rural atmosphere as were some of the mining villages. There were of course the slag heaps, mine shafts and fiery furnaces, but we did have Little Pant and on the west slope was the Trevethin Wood. Rising steeply to three hundred feet, it harboured a variety of trees in straggling abundance rarely seen today, now that shaded green armies of spruce and fir stand rigidly aligned on every hill.

There were boughs to swing upon, trunks to scale, nuts to eat and huts to build. In the undergrowth there were rabbits to be tracked, nests to discover and secret hiding places. To the village kids it was paradise, a natural garden with bees and butterflies, shade and sunshine and, if one wanted, peace and isolation.

But in stark contrast, as if to emphasise the divide between good and evil, between it and the village ran the Avon Llwyd, the Grey River.

Born fresh and free at the valley head, in its travels it absorbed the trappings of the community's rejection as displayed by bottles and tins, lumpy sacks tightly secured, assorted garments, dead sheep, old tyres and slimy, unidentifiable objects that floated along on a cushion of grey-black scum.

There was no life in the Grey River in those days.

Any natural movement, other than the turgid swirling

of its pockmarked, evil surface, was confined to the large grey rats that scurried over its black shores, happy in the knowledge that their environment was of such a filthy nature that there was no competition for the right of possession.

And yet, this Stygian watercourse, like Little Pant, also played a part in moulding my ambitions towards a veterinary life.

To cross the river there was a bridge at Cwm Frwdd Halt and another, about a mile or so downstream, at the Foundry. It made a pleasant walk after Chapel to cross into the wood at one bridge and out at the other, returning via the road.

But to the boys of the village there was only *one* way to the Trevethin Wood: across the Boggy Pipe.

Where it came from, where it went and what its purpose was I didn't know — even to this day I'm not too sure — but it was black, fifty feet long, three feet in diameter and it traversed the river. On each bank, two brick pillars eight feet high, topped with smooth concrete, stabilised either end of the pipe and supported the black iron girder that ran beneath it right across the murky divide.

At two-foot intervals, raised iron hoops clamped the girth of the pipe to the girder.

In the unlikely event of anyone being foolish enough to try to climb upon the pillars, rows of razor-sharp, multicoloured fragments of broken bottles had been embedded in the concrete to foil the attempt.

As if this wasn't sufficient to deter such a maniacal act, barbed wire had been wound in profusion around the front of the pillar and the first three feet of the pipe, to make the passage from pillar to pipe an act beyond the comprehension of any rational mind.

It was this pipe that the village boys regularly traversed in order to get to the Trevethin Wood.

To the accomplished it presented no problem. To others it was a void in the happiness of youthful experience and a barrier to full involvement and participation in the joys of the Trevethin Wood. When gangs crossed the pipe, the weak had to run up- or downstream to the bridges. Breathlessly we would stumble through the trees to the other side, eager to join up with the mob. But by the time contact had been made, nuts had been devoured, blackberries consumed, trees booked and friendships struck.

If you didn't go across the Boggy Pipe it was useless. You missed out on everything.

There were two reasons why I had never attempted to cross the Boggy Pipe. One was that Mother had forbidden it, and the other, that I was very, very scared.

Many was the night I had attempted to cross it in my mind as I lay in bed. But even in the secure and friendly confines of my room, I could not bring myself mentally to finish the course. I saw myself isolated for ever, clinging to the middle, the waters of the Avon Llwyd sucking at my feet, while dead sheep, multicoloured rats, green glass bottles and slimy things spun in a devil's merry-go-round beneath.

How I envied the Boggy Crossers. How I watched, spellbound with admiration, as a First-Timer clambered down the far pillar onto the foreign bank amid the whoops and cheers of his pals.

There was no doubt that in Abergranog village in those days the supreme embodiment of all that was brave and bold, daring and defiant, adventurous in one's character; the act that separated men from boys; the finite achievement that put the valiant beyond the mundane flow of daily events — was to cross the Boggy Pipe!

That's how I saw it, anyway, when I was in Class Three at Abergranog Council School. And I knew I would have to do it some time.

There was more than one method of crossing. The Pipe could be Ridden, Sided or — and this was the ultimate — it could be Walked.

In every case the method of access was similar.

Footholds had been created in the brickwork by the Boggy Crossers and the glassware had been levelled in small patches at the top to allow careful placement of knees for the two-foot shuffle through the barbed wire and onto the pipe.

Periodically, the Council would send someone to tighten up the wire barricades, but a little work by the older Boggy Crossers soon widened the strands so that it was fairly easy to crawl through.

As the pipe was about one foot below the top of the pillars, it was necessary to ease one's legs down the side and then drop onto the top of it, steadying the balance as one landed. This was the most difficult part.

And all the time the stinking waters ran beneath.

From then on, the choice of position depended upon the method adopted. Riding was a series of jerks astride the pipe, easing over the raised securing hoops as they were reached. As the pipe was about fifty feet long, it took over one hundred movements, plus ten lifts over the hoops. From the point of safety, that was the best method, but physically it was extremely punishing, bringing tears to the eyes and bruises and swellings in little private places.

It was therefore well worth graduating to Siding, which was far less damaging to the anatomy. This entailed shuffling alongside the body of the pipe with both feet on the the lip of the girder below and with arms and chest over the top. One had to be tall enough to reach over to balance safely, but it was much quicker and about twenty movements got you there.

But of all the Boggy Crossers, the supremos were the Walkers. They were of exceptional flair and undeniably brave, for they not only walked across the top of the pipe but even returned from halfway; some could stand on one leg, and Felix Pugh, so rumour had it, had actually done a hand stand, although I had never seen it.

The spur to my attempt came one morning at school when Wendel Weekes announced: 'Saturday morning I'm goin' to cross the Boggy!'

I was staggered.

Wendel was two months my junior, smaller and in my opinion far more timid than I. At once Wendel surpassed me in the attention he attracted from several others who overheard. Cries of admiration at his intended feat came from around and, although I added my support, I felt sick at the thought of his possible achievement.

My time had come. I had to cross the Boggy before him.

It was difficult to concentrate on the sex life of the butterfly that afternoon, and I twice got the thick end of Miss Webb's tongue for not paying attention. But at five to four, the bell rang and, like a pack of Pavlov's dogs, a response was immediate with a shuffling of feet, closing of books, banging of desks and murmurs of relief sweeping the class. It was hometime — but not for me.

Down the tiled stairway, into the cloakroom to grab my cap, out through the playground, the gates, the road.

'Where you goin'?' shouted Wendel. 'Wait for me.'

But I was away, running fast. Down the Incline, past the Rising Sun, the Railway Gulley, across Hubbard's Patch and on.

On to the Boggy Pipe.

I was drained of mental and physical energy as I approached the river bank. Exhausted, I fell to my knees.

Could Scyrion have felt more humble as he viewed the Mount of Zenat? Or Peachley, from his small canoe, have prayed harder as he drew towards the mighty Falls of Wardour? Did those brave boyhood heroes blink at fate and, biting on their lips, drive forward to their doom . . . or stand and shiver in the thinning air, knees weak and schoolboy cap in hand?

I couldn't let my champions down.

The pillars were easy, mainly because the footholds were well worn and my mental rehearsals of previous nights had been so thorough. In seconds I had scaled the wall, negotiated the broken glass with only minor abrasions and was soon astride the stony prominence that overlooked the insert of the pipe.

Now came the most difficult part. Dropping onto the pipe.

The principle was to ease the body downwards, taking the weight on the palms of the hands.

The launch was the worst moment. Below, the black forbidding tube that seemed to stretch away into the distance, never ending. Beneath, the swirling, stinking waters of the Avon Llwyd.

Even little boys, within the confines of their inexperience, can be great heroes. Small may be the feats. Pointless in comparison. Silly. Futile. Little games. But all the physiology of gland and muscle, all the nervous energy that swims along the stream from brain to tissue, vies with the surge of any athlete's exertion or the steel of courage in the field.

If my grasp hadn't slipped, I would probably have gone home at that moment. But it did — and I fell sharply onto the Boggy Pipe.

As if connected to an electrical impulse, I started to go through the humpy, jerky, crutch-savaging motions that I had seen the proven Boggy Crossers do. And, to my surprise, it wasn't so difficult and I found I was making good progress. Even the first ring was no problem and I was actually beginning to enjoy Riding the Boggy. It was so wide that the wicked waters were obscured from direct view. The far pillar was still quite distant, but straight ahead. I was on my way.

Hump. Jerk. Hump. Jerk.

I was well into the second half, when I saw its head appear above the concrete prominence facing me. It rose slowly and uncertainly, ears pricked, eyes shining, and, as I sat perfectly still, it came into full view. Then, standing erect, silhouetted against the sky, just a ginger and white handful of fluff, it opened its jaws and gave vent to a weak: 'Miaow!'

My passage blocked, I stared in anguish at the little

bundle as it perched on the pillar edge. Then, to my horror, it gave another squeaky 'Miaow', jumped onto the pipe and started to walk towards me.

'Go back, little cat!' I cried. 'Out the way!'

But the little cat just squeaked again, its tail a-quiver as, pad by pad, on it came.

Unsteadily I raised my right hand, waved it in short jerks and hissed through my teeth:

'SSSsssss! Shoo! Back, cat! Go home!'

At this it stopped, just out of my reach, sat down, cocked its head on one side and sort of smiled and started to clean its paws.

'Little cat,' I pleaded, 'go back! Please! You're tiny, I'm big. You turn round an' go back, there's a good puss.'

I raised my eyebrows expectantly and the beads of cold sweat ran sideways down my forehead. It was then that I knew I was frightened and I started to panic.

The kitten seemed to sense my fear and stood up, squeaking an acknowledgement of my request, its tiny pink tongue brushing its damp nose.

It was moving, it was going to turn.

To my relief, round it went to face the far pillar.

'Good boy, cat!' I shouted.

At that, it turned round again and came towards me. It seemed bigger and more purposeful, it was striding at me.

'Go back!' I screamed. 'I'm frightened!'

I took off my cap and waved it forward.

I never pushed it ... honest! I never even meant to touch it, but the movement momentarily unbalanced it. The fluffy little body twisted unevenly, thin claws scrabbing at the black-tarred surface. Still its tail quivered, but it was too far over. Pink tongue showing, it opened its mouth, but no sound came and, like a leaf dropping, it seemed to float gently downwards and was suddenly lost in the foaming black bubbles of the river below.

I made no sound either, no breath or movement of any sort, and my mind became blank as, numbed with shock, I sat upon the Boggy Pipe.

A slight giddiness came over me and I lengthened my gaze from the spot where the little body had disappeared to further downstream.

A small muddy peninsula jutted into the murky waters about twenty yards below the bridge, trapping a conglomeration of branches, tin cans and mouldy sacking beneath a decaying tree. At first I thought it was a rat moving, but rats had long leathery tails, not little spiky ones that stuck up. Wet it was and squeaking as it clambered into the partly submerged branches.

The little cat was alive.

All feelings of shock and guilt fled from me. Adrenalin filled my blood and I humped and jerked for the far pillar, shouting:

'Wait, little cat! I'm coming!'

I don't remember scaling the far pillar, or the broken glass, or the barbed wire. In no time at all I was there, within a yard of the little cat.

But it was a vital yard across that black frothy divide.

I lay on my belly and reached. I tried my foot but couldn't touch bottom. I sat and stretched with my legs until they were both in the filthy water and soaking wet. I searched frantically for a stick, pole, rope, hook — anything.

Anything . . . but there was nothing to help.

The little cat was still clambering about amid the loose branches. If only I could have reached it, I could have pulled it inshore.

I searched the area again — and then I found it: a piece of barbed wire, cut off at some time from the pillar. Just the thing. I straightened it out and raced back to the scene.

It was long enough to reach the floating branches and its barbs hooked into the wood. Slowly I drew the mass toward me.

'Just you hold on tight, boyo,' I called, 'an' 'ew'll be safe.'

And as if it knew, the little cat stopped moving and squeaked in reply.

The drag was getting heavier and I felt myself being drawn forward with the weight.

I must have been just a foot away and on the point of grabbing the nearest twigs with my right hand, when the wire lost its grip and the whole lot swished back like a spring, catapulting the little mite into midstream.

Tears of frustration and grief welled into my eyes; I watched, helplessly, as it was washed away. It bobbed and spun in the choppy water for about five yards. Then suddenly, a rolling eddy sucked it backwards and deposited it on a flat stone only inches from the opposite bank.

There was no decision, question or hesitation in my action. Scyrion and Peachley both, would surely have applauded, for I was back across the Boggy Pipe and down river to that flat stone, scooping the little cat into my arms and sobbing with relief and joy. I cuddled the sodden, stinking little thing under my jersey and turned for home.

The parting glance I gave the Boggy Pipe just registered the line of wet footprints along its top, but their significance escaped me until later.

I had saved the little cat. That was enough for now.

I told Mother everything — I always did — never could keep anything from her. She didn't go mad, and when I brought the little cat from under my jersey, I thought she was going to cry.

'You naughty boy,' she said, but without any scolding in her voice, as she took the shivering little body from me. 'You could have drowned yourself.'

'Can we keep him?' I asked, eagerly, the trials of the afternoon now far behind.

'It might belong to someone,' she said, stroking its wet coat.

'If no one says, can we?' I pleaded.

'Well, if no one says, I suppose so,' she replied.

And I knew no one would, for in Abergranog, even in those hard times, there were two commodities that were ever plentiful. One was rhubarb — and the other, kittens.

Now-a-days, the modern terminology for a pet is a companion animal, and if ever there was a companion, that little cat was one to me.

Boggy I called him — after all, what else could he have been?

The ginger tom never left my side, except when I was at school. Then, he would wait at the bottom of the lane and, seeing me approach, would stand up, stretch luxuriously, then spring up the wall and delicately pick his way towards me, flourishing his fluffy tail and purring like a motor boat. When alongside, I would stop, he would climb onto my shoulders and home we would go.

At week-ends we went across the Boggy Pipe – it held no fears any more, for I could walk it as good as the rest and even put my hands in my pockets. Boggy would follow closely behind.

We would go a little downstream from the pipe, just below where I had fished him out. He would sit like a terrier on the edge of the black mud while I beat the bank with a stick. With any luck a rat would come scurrying out of the long grass and Boggy, who was now developing into a fine, agile creature, would dive at it like a tiger. He was mustard when it came to rats and never lost a contest.

Sometimes we would climb up into the wood and I would lie upon my back and watch the clouds scudding over the top of the hill, as if glad to be free of our grubby patch. Boggy would sit, patiently staring into a clump of undergrowth. Suddenly he would pounce and, after a bit of commotion, emerge with a shrew, which he would proudly lay at my feet.

One summer afternoon, while I lay deep in inconsequential meditation, a scream of earsplitting pitch seared the air. I sat up gasping. It was a desperate childlike cry, urgent yet pitiful. I looked down the path in front of me to see Boggy approaching, proudly carrying a young rabbit in his mouth.

Rats and shrews brought no remorse to my heart, but the cry of the rabbit was so uncannily human that I shouted:

'Let him go. Let him go, Boggy.'

But Boggy stood firm and growled in a most aggressive manner. I leaped forward and grabbed at the rabbit. Boggy reluctantly released it, then backed off a few paces, eyes flashing angrily — I had never known him show such hostility towards me before. Still growling, he wove from side to side, flicking the tip of his tail and never taking his eyes off me. For a moment I thought he was going to spring, then he turned about and walked slowly away.

The young rabbit had stopped squealing and lay shivering in my hands. It didn't appear to have any serious injuries, so I waded into the undergrowth and let it go. When I got back to the path, Boggy was waiting for me. I picked him up and stroked his soft ginger coat and he started to purr deeply. Then we went home and I carried him all the way.

That night I lay awake thinking about the incident. I could still see the aggression in Boggy's eyes and knew that at that moment there had been no companionship — I had been his enemy. I think that taught me to respect animals and appreciate their natural instincts, although, to me, Boggy was still a grand cat and quite entitled to his opinion.

On Sundays, when we went to Chapel, I would lock Boggy in the shed. I had done this ever since the fateful morning he turned up during the service.

Our chapel was the standard Baptist design, with bottom-aching, oakstained pews on the ground floor and the deacon's seats and pulpit at the head. Upstairs was the gallery, railed off by a wrought iron screen, with choir seats behind and, at the front, a green and gold pipe organ. The younger Miss Prowle performed upon the ancient instrument, hidden from view by a red woollen curtain that hung from big brass rings on a long rail. She took the whole thing very seriously.

I remember the event as clearly as if it were yesterday.

The Reverend Deri Jones was praying, everyone was bowed and I was looking down, busily counting the knot holes in the wooden floor. The Reverend Deri was a most impressive figure with a shock of white hair, wing collar, frock coat and pince-nez. For me, these glasses provided the highlight of the service, for the Reverend Deri never removed them by hand; when he had finished reading or singing he would just tweak his nose and they would fall towards the floor, happily saved by a black cord that attached them to his lapel.

When the great man prayed he would close his eyes tightly and turn his face to the ceiling. He would pray for everything and anything in a deep monotone, and sometimes it lasted for half an hour. The effect was quite soporific for most adults, but I found it rather boring.

That morning he had been going for about ten minutes and was as far as the missionaries in Borneo, when a high-pitched scream came from behind the organ curtain. The fabric moved violently and suddenly the younger Miss Prowle shot out from behind it, hatless and dishevelled. Everyone looked up, but the Reverend Deri kept on going.

Then, I noticed the fringe of the curtain rise up in one corner and a small head appeared — a small ginger head. It was Boggy. And that wasn't all: in his mouth he held a bunch of short feathers, the same colour as the younger Miss Prowle's hat.

Slowly he emerged from beneath the curtain, then hopped over the empty seats and sprang onto the gallery rail whence he eyed the congregation suspiciously — and all the time the Reverend Deri kept on praying.

My father, who was sitting alongside, gave me a rather bewildered look, then he covered his face with his hand and bowed his head reverently — but I think he was hiding a smile.

Up until then, nobody knew whose cat it was, but then

Boggy spied me and all was up.

He leaped from the gallery rail onto the pulpit and walked across in front of the Reverend Deri, still with the feathers in his mouth. Then down the steps he came, on up the aisle and turned in to our pew where he dropped his trophy at my feet.

'It's Boggy,' I whispered to my father. But he didn't answer, just nodded and kept his face covered.

I scooped up my cat and, with head down, made for the door. As I reached it the Reverend Deri was uttering his final 'Aaa-men'; due to his communion with the Almighty, he had remained oblivious of the whole commotion.

The repercussions were milder than I had expected. My Auntie Min, who was a dressmaker and had two cats of her own, offered to repair the younger Miss Prowle's hat for nothing, on condition that Boggy was confined to the shed on Sundays. Dad said it must never happen again, but I did detect a twinkle in his eye when he told me.

For two years Boggy and I were great pals, then one day he went missing.

A feeling of uneasiness came over me when he wasn't on the wall after school. I ran home and searched and called. I asked all about and missed my tea. When it grew dark I became very worried.

'Perhaps he's gone off on a jaunt,' said Dad. 'Tom cats often do.'

But I couldn't believe it of Boggy.

I didn't sleep much that night, my mind constantly working over all his haunts and habits. Then a thought struck me — perhaps he was in the Trevethin Wood. I knew he went there sometimes when I was in school because Tom Ellis, the woodman, had told me.

At first light I went down to Mr Ellis' cottage. He was shaving in the back yard and stood, great hairy shaving brush in hand, as I approached.

'Have you seen Boggy, Mr Ellis?' I asked, urgently.

The old man blew the lather from his lips.

'Boggy?' he questioned.

'My cat. He's ginger and white — you've seen him before.'

'Oh. That cat.' He tickled up the lather with his brush and ducked his head to glance into a piece of cracked mirror glass upon the wall. In fact, there were all types of oddments on Mr Ellis' wall. Everything from tools to tyres, horseshoes to hurricane lamps and metal pieces, with ratchets and coils of fine wire.

The woodman shook his head and reached for his cut-throat razor, opening it expertly with one hand and holding it up so that its blade flashed coldly in the early morning sun.

'Haven't seen him for a long time,' he said.

'Do you think he might be in the wood?'

'Might be,' he replied, turning away, and with a deft sweep of his hand started to strip the lather from his face with the razor.

I still had time before school to make a quick search, so out across Hubbard's Patch I sped and on to the Boggy Pipe.

I was half way across when I saw him. Not walking towards me as he did when we first met, but lying motionless at the foot of the far pillar.

When I got to him his eyes were open and he weakly parted his lips, but made no sound, neither did he move. Then I noticed the piece of wood just behind him; it had been cut from a tree and pointed with a knife. Running from it was a short cord joined to a thin piece of wire similar to the coils seen hanging on Mr Ellis' wall. The wire disappeared into Boggy's coat and when I picked him up, the stick and cord came as well.

He was so limp and lifeless, he just hung in my arms, and as the tears welled up I held him tightly to my chest. Boggy was breathing, but only very gently, and cradling him in front of me I carried him back along the pipe.

When I got to Mr Ellis' cottage he was at his gate, as if he was expecting me.

'I've found him, but he's hurt,' I sobbed. 'Look at him.'

Mr Ellis took Boggy from me, carried him into his tiny kitchen and, pushing aside the cups and plates, laid him on the table. Then he went to a drawer and came back with a pair of pliers. Parting Boggy's ginger fur, he snipped through the wire.

'What is it, Mr Ellis?' I asked, as he unwound the thing from the limp form and threw it in a corner.

'For rabbits,' he said, 'not cats. But he got caught in it.'

I didn't understand the implication as I do now as a country vet. For to live in the countryside is to accept country ways and to understand that the balance of nature is maintained, often in cruel mode. The childlike screams of the rabbit, the lethal dive of the hawk, the fluttering panic in the hen coop when the fox appears. But when your cat drags itself home with a wire snare cutting into its skin and its hind limbs paralysed, it becomes unacceptable.

A snare is a braided wire running noose. The noose is spread in a rabbit track, usually in a gap in hedge or undergrowth, and pegged securely and unobtrusively alongside the natural run. There is no distinction between its victims. Silently, it awaits rabbit, fox or cat on the scent.

Designed to garrotte — that is the easy way out — the wretched animal can also be trapped around the belly, as was Boggy. Or by the hind limbs or just one leg, and the agony is unimaginable. It has been known for a fox to bite off a portion of its own limb in an attempt to escape, leaving but a vestige of a trophy for the hunter.

I was fortunate that I didn't fully comprehend the significance at that time.

'Will he get better, Mr Ellis?' I asked.

The old man's newly shaven, craggy face softened and he looked down at the little cat; with his large rough hands he gently stroked the ginger coat and shook his head.

I couldn't believe it — I wouldn't believe it.

''Is back is broke,' he said. ''E'll never walk again.'

I tried to be brave. I tried hard for a good minute. Then I

couldn't hold it and sobbed uncontrollably.

Eventually, I calmed down and Mr Ellis put his hand on my shoulder.

'You go home,' he said. 'I'll see to Boggy.'

'What are you going to do, Mr Ellis?' I asked, through my tears.

'Take his pain away,' said the old man. 'It's the best thing.'

He saw me to his gate and, as I closed it, I turned towards him. There was one question I had to ask:

'Was it your wire, Mr Ellis?'

'Go home, son,' said the old man gently, without answering my question. 'I'll come and see your father tonight.'

He did come and see Father, and three weeks later he turned up again with a little grey kitten which he gave to me and which I called Pip. Since those days I've had a lot of cats: there was Smoky, Max, Crispin and Tarquin, to name but a few. But they never did and never will mean the same to me as Boggy. I think it's mainly because through him I learned to respect animals, know what company they can be and understand now-a-days how my clients feel when their cat has to be put down.

And it's also because of Boggy that I've hated snares ever since.

*   *   *

If there was any other part of Abergranog village that contributed to my feelings for animals it was the Park.

The Park had been a small estate, left to the mining community by a local benefactor. A green oasis set amid the drab stonework of the village, it was surrounded for the most part by a high wall and was about four acres in all. A red ash path had been laid through the centre, circling a large clock on an iron stand that was a memorial to a local doctor and told a different time on each of its four sides. The entrances, of which there were two, were guarded by large iron gates, one at the Factory Lane end and the other leading onto Bowen's Pitch. Just off the path at the Factory Lane was the Shelter, a small openfronted building with lavatories at either side.

The big house had long been demolished, but the lawns and rose gardens remained intact, as did the African Hut. This mysterious structure was actually the summer house belonging to the old residence and took its nickname from the fact that it was a black wooden construction with a conical straw roof, situated beneath a large willow at the end of the garden. Adding to the tribal atmosphere was the fact that the old men of the village spent most of the daytime inside, festooned in acrid smoke from the shag and twist of the day.

The fug was fresh air to their shrunken, pneumoconiotic lungs and stimulated wheezing laughter, crawing, spitting and much stamping of sticks.

The smoke was often so intense that it could be seen easing its way through the straw, as if the place was on fire, for the only ventilation — and light for that matter — came through a small doorway at the front.

It was all in the care of Parky, Ernie Brewer, a mousy little man who manicured the shrubs and roses and wrestled with the great clattering mower that swathed the lawns in shaded lines. Ernie's new-mown grass was as nectar. In those days the smell of Park grass and 4711 Eau-de-Cologne, which my mother used, were my favourite aromas.

Park sounds, too, I remember. Creaking swings, flushing lavatories, the old mower and kids shouting. But the one more abiding memory of mystery, intrigue, sound, smell and even colour, was that of the Co-op Slaughter-house which was next to the children's playground.

If you swung high enough, you got regular fleeting glimpses through the gaps in the shutters. Always the floor was wet; sometimes red wet, sometimes brown, sometimes green. Wellington boots you could see and the bottom of red rubber aprons. Once I saw a little calf lying on its side, very still.

But only once.

Sweeping, sweeping, the sound of someone constantly sweeping; whoever worked the bass broom in the Co-op Slaughterhouse worked hard. Whistling and singing I remember, bleating and lowing, the clang of metal chains and sharp cracks, like fireworks exploding.

In summer it smelt terrible: rich, sickly sweet and throat retching; but still we watched, swatting the big blue flies that sunned themselves on the brick wall. In the narrow gully by the side of the roundabout they kept the offal: great, glistening cow stomachs, mounds of partly digested fodder and animal guts in a thousand convolutions.

From the road between the buildings, when the wooden sliding door was open, you could see them killing sheep.

The word would spread about the Park and we kids would crowd, with morbid fascination, compelled to watch, hypnotised by the spectacle.

Two men with caps on worked side by side, one of them Parky's brother. Periodically they disappeared into the gloom of the building, to return, carrying a struggling woolly bundle which they dumped in a trough and plunged at with a knife.

The legs would thrash wildly as the victim's life gurgled away, and in no time at all, with an iron hook between its jaws, it was a lump of meat suspended on a rail, alongside its unfortunate fellows.

*   *   *

I often wonder how much the experiences of my youthful days in Abergranog guided me into my present way of life.

Was it Old Thundertits and that day at Little Pant, and the unforgettable feeling of newborn life in her offspring's foot? Was it the joy and sadness of having a pet like Boggy? Or was it pity for those poor dead sheep hanging on the rail and that little calf lying on its side, ever so still?

Perhaps it was a mix of all of this, and even the smell of

Ernie Brewer's new mown grass, that made me leave Abergranog to settle eventually in Herefordshire as a country vet.

Two

As Miss Webb might have put it:

'If a crow was to fly, say, over Trevethin Wood, around Abergavenny and up through Pendulas to Ledingford, much quicker it would be than going via Glasgow, wouldn't it?'

And, of course it would have been, but Glasgow, and in particular the University, was my way of going to Ledingford. In retrospect, it was a very formative way and my valley mind, like the narrow mountain roads, was broadened into motorway proportions.

In due course I passed for grammar school, played Rugby, sang in the choir, acted in the school play and worked hard at physics and chemistry. But it was biology that I enjoyed most. No need for calculators or computers, for thought was relatively uncluttered. Those were the days of dogfish, frog and rabbit; of basic dissection and labelled diagrams, in a simple quest to find out how things worked. This simplicity was invaluable in moulding my future feelings for animals, helping to avoid the danger that modern methods and technology can spread of regarding living things as insensitive units of production or exploitation.

National Service was a legacy of the War, and unless one was able to secure one of the few places allocated to school leavers, it was the army first.

I was very fortunate in being granted a place at Glasgow.

There were seven university colleges teaching veterinary science at the time. London and Edinburgh were the oldest and most popular, then followed Glasgow and Liverpool, the two newest being Bristol and Cambridge. There was also a college in Dublin that I once visited on a Rugby tour. We spent most of the trip at the Guinness Brewery and at the time I thought how grand it would have been to study there.

But it was Glasgow that would have me and Glasgow I accepted. I didn't know what I was going into — and they certainly didn't know what they were getting. But it worked out all right for both of us in the end.

When I arrived at Central Station on that foggy October night, it was like entering a vast oil drum — dark, smelly and smoky.

Abergranog was sometimes dark and smelly, and often the wicked Welsh mist came down, embalming the valley in its cold, invisible breath. Yet, when it parted, hedgerows and trees would ghost silently into view. But the Glasgow fog was green, evil and penetrating and when it parted — there was just more fog.

Suddenly I missed the Trevethin Wood and Little Pant, the Park and even the Avon Llwyd. As the taxi rattled over the cobbled streets and bodged across the tram lines I spied Glaswegian bodies shuffling through the gloom, I felt rather lonely and wondered how that environment could ever mould me into a country vet.

But over the next five years I was to discover a Celtic warmth and companionship in that city and to come to understand how Sir Harry Lauder could sing with such feeling 'I belong tae Glasgae'.

I found my digs and the following day saw the University at Gilmorehill. As I walked through Kelvingrove Park, the frostchilled mist gradually cleared and the towers and pinnacles of the great building took form. As I drew closer, the grand symmetry of its design became apparent, a monument to five hundred years of industry and learning.

The awe-inspiring sight lifted my depression and I knew that I had come to the right place.

Five years was and still is a long time to study for a career and be supported to achieve it. Financial assistance was not as generous as it is today and many parents, my own included, made considerable sacrifices to keep their offspring at university. Student life was poor but happy.

But the long course did have one peculiar advantage, in that the student not only learned to be a veterinary surgeon, but gradually grew into one.

In the very beginning, however, the incentive to join the profession and the urge to ease animal pain and suffering could, despite even the deepest enthusiasm, be severely shaken by the anatomy classes. The first time I entered the Dissection Hall I was silently shocked.

I knew that, in order to discover how animals were built, they were best studied by taking them apart, piece by piece. After all, I'd done it with dogfish, frog and rabbit. But I wasn't prepared for the sight of large animal cadavers arranged in peculiar poses like plasticine models, grey, stodgy and in various stages of undress.

There were horses, skinned and lying on their backs, feet pointed rigidly to the ceiling; cows of indeterminable breed stripped of muscle so that the light shone through gaunt frames; from assorted tables sheep and pig heads gazed forlornly into space and, at the far end of the Hall, was positioned a large preserving tank — when I cautiously peered over the rim I discovered it to be full of failed greyhounds. Above, ran great gantries with pulley chains to assist the manipulation of the bodies, while fixed upon the walls were gaily coloured gazetteers of nerve pathways, bloodvessel patterns and bone structures. The whole room, though brightly lit, had a stifling atmosphere tainted with the pungent aroma of formalin that made the eyes smart, the stomach uneasy and the palms moist.

Becoming a vet was taking a bit of getting used to, but in due course I became acclimatised and involved in tracing the intricate pathways of arteries and veins, following nerve supplies and locating the attachments of ligaments and muscles; I came to regard specimens, like the horse, as a system of pulleys that ate hay, rather than a dead body.

There was much to learn about other species as well as the horse. Cow, pig, sheep, dog, cat and even fowl were studied. This comparative anatomy made me envy the human medical students who, with some slight variations, always had their specimens with them. I felt this made it much easier to appreciate kidney pain, indigestion or skin rashes in their patients than to understand how a cow feels when its five stomachs are aching, which joint hurts in a lame horse or what an itch in fur, wool or feathers feels like. I often wondered if cows got headaches and whether it would be possible to prove it.

*   *   *

So far I had seen no sick or ailing animals. In fact, the pre-clinical years were entirely devoted to the study of normality, for without that, the abnormal could in no way be truly appreciated. But if I had learnt anything up until then, it was about the intricate balance and harmony that exists in every living being, even in such humble creatures as the barnyard fowl.

And it was in the barnyards of the Vale of Usk that I spent my summer vacations during those first years. It was most essential to obtain as much background and experience in agriculture as possible, and working on the farms was the best way to get it.

One of my most memorable experiences actually occurred in a barnyard, on the very first day I started work at Brynheulog Farm.

Brynheulog, which when translated means 'the hill where the sun shines', was aptly named. It consisted of a compact group of whitewashed stone buildings, situated upon a rising fold of ground at the foot of the roundshouldered Blorenge Mountain that overlooked Abergavenny.

It was a family farm, running a small mixed dairy herd, pigs, sheep, ducks and chickens, and growing enough corn and roots to feed the stock. There was an orchard with both sweet and sour fruit, a pond with coots and a pine wood full of soft cooing wood-pigeons. The farmhouse was lowbeamed and cosy, the dairy flagstoned and cool, and the fascinating lavatory was a small hut at the bottom of the garden. Fascinating to me because it had two seats — suggesting a joint venture I found difficult to imagine.

David Morgan, a small intense Welshman, had taken me on as general hand for the summer.

'Just goin' off on the round,' he said curtly, through the van window, when I met him in the lane. For every Monday he took cream, eggs, potatoes and other produce up to Llanavon at the top of the next valley, where he sold his wares from door to door. 'You go and give Dicko a hand. He's my man an' he's putting the barn ready — he knows you're coming.' He gave a wave and revved the engine; the old Austin spluttered and jerked off down the track.

I faced Brynheulog, the sun sparkling on its white-washed walls, and, with a rich mixture of country aromas in my nostrils, set forth to find Dicko.

I had no idea where the barnyard was, but after going through the cowhouse, into the roothouse and out by the stables, I found it. It was cobbled and part covered in seeded corn, and on a neatly stacked midden in the far corner about twenty Rhode Island hens squabbled and scratched with great vigour. To the left, a Dutch barn ran in continuation with the farm buildings, one of the bays still stacked with the previous year's fodder.

Apart from the hens and a wall-eyed collie dog eyeing me suspiciously through the bars of the gate, there was no sign of life.

'Dicko!' I shouted. 'Are you there?'

I stood for a few minutes awaiting a response. Then, I shouted again.

The second time, I did get a reaction.

'D'yer know anything about chickens, Mr Vet?' a voice bellowed from above.

Startled, I looked upwards and stood back a pace to

discover a round, red face peering down at me from the gap between the high stack and the barn roof.

'D'yer know anything about chickens?' the face repeated, beginning to deepen in colour.

'I've done some anatomy,' I responded rather weakly, still a bit confused by the turn of events.

'Wha's wrong with this, then?' asked the red face, and dropped an egg from his lofty position down to me. Instinctively I cupped my hands and caught it, the shell shattering in a dozen pieces, and from the mess came the foulest smell I have ever encountered. I stood there, rigid, as the green-black, stinking contents oozed malevolently between my fingers.

'It's rotten!' I shouted, half choking.

'Right!' roared the red face, in a gale of laughter. 'Right yer be! That must be a hell of a fine college you be at!'

I threw the egg in the midden and plunged both hands deep into the water trough. I was livid and clenched my fists — whoever owned the red face was in trouble.

'I'm comin' down,' came a shout, still full of raucous laughter.

I moved to the corner of the stack, burning with anger, poising myself ready to take revenge.

Then the Red Face emerged.

He was shorter than I, but that was my only advantage, for he was built like an ox; his cheery red face, topped by a hayseed-covered cap, ran directly into his broad shoulders, which could have supported the Llanellen Bridge. About forty, hair flowed luxuriant from his open-necked flannel shirt and his moleskin trousers were gathered at his solid midriff by a wide, black leather belt, joined by a powerful brass buckle.

Had this not been enough to make me reconsider my original intention, the thickness of his forearms and the breadth of his horny hands soon made up my mind. My anger quickly subsided.

'No offence, Mr Vet. Just a lark. Dicko Jeeps is the name. Now, try a drop o' this.' And he thrust a small earthenware jar into my hands. 'Don' be frit of it, it ain't rotten,' he said, his face still wreathed in a smile. 'I won't pull yer leg no more.'

It was good cider in the little jar, and not the last I was to have from it, for that summer I worked alongside the genial countryman and learned much about country ways.

One morning I found Dicko mixing up an evil-looking potion in an old jug. It smelled quite intoxicating and Dicko stirred away with the obvious delight of an ancient witch mixing a brew.

'Us be 'avin' a party tonight. You comin'?' he asked, jovially.

'No thanks,' I replied. 'It looks awful.'

'Old Jasper's bound up,' explained Dicko. 'So I'm makin' a drop o' "special" for 'im. By rights you ought to be seein' ter this, Mr Vet,' he winked, broadly, then stirred the mixture with renewed vigour.

Jasper was the Large White boar, a great, mean, hairy creature who lived in a part of the stable building, just off the yard.

'Won't eat or drink an's got real miserable,' said Dicko. 'Right off 'is jim-jam, too, 'e is — if yer know what I means.' He gave another wicked wink.

'Whatever is in it?' I asked, as the alcoholic aroma wafted towards me.

'Salts an' cider, with a little bit of castor oil. 'An' if that don't shift 'im, nothin' will!'

'I can believe that,' I agreed. 'But if he isn't eating or drinking, how are you going to give it to him?'

'How are *we* goin' ter give it to 'im, Mr Vet,' said Dicko, rubbing his hands. 'Bring that jow'line and I'll get me boot.'

I picked up the thin ploughrope and made my way out to the stable where Dicko joined me, carefully setting down the jugful of medicine and an old riding boot with the toe cut away.

Jasper lay grunting unconcernedly in the straw in one

corner, as Dicko explained his plan.

'I slips the noose of the jow'line round 'is snout an' throws it over that beam,' he said, pointing to a rough oak strut running under the roof. 'You catch it an' pull up, hard as you can, then 'e'll back up against the wall an' I can stuff the boot down 'is gullet an' pour the jollop through the toe, an' Bob's yer uncle!'

It sounded straightforward enough, so long as Jasper was in agreement. He soon showed he wasn't as the noose tightened around his snout, and leaped to his feet complaining loudly. I grabbed the loose end that Dicko hurled over the beam and pulled for all I was worth. Jasper fought and wriggled, causing the beam to creak ominously.

''Old 'im steady!' shouted Dicko, advancing upon the great foaming jaws with the boot in one hand and jug in the other. But Jasper would have none of it. Eventually, he gave in to the rope and stood still, but whenever Dicko touched his mouth with the lip of the boot, he shook his head violently.

'No good from the front,' said Dicko. 'I'll get behind his head an' pull it in from the back.'

'Are you sure you can manage it?' I asked, doubtfully. 'Sounds a bit dangerous.'

'Seen it done afore,' retorted Dicko. 'Jus' you 'old that rope tight. I'll show yer summat to tell 'em back at that college of your'n.'

With boot and jug in hand, he straddled the boar's neck and leaned forward. Jasper squatted a few inches to take Dicko's weight, then pushed robustly against the rope.

'Don' yer let go now!' gasped Dicko, trying to keep his balance.

'I won't!' I shouted.

Then, suddenly, an evil thought entered my mind and the smell of rotten eggs came flooding back. For there was Dicko, who had had such fun at my expense on my first day at Brynheulog, now sitting with his back to me, astride a great pig. And the only thing stopping him from going for one hell of a ride was the rope — which I was holding.

I was savouring the power in my possession, when Jasper made a sudden jerk and my arms fell as the rope went slack. I stumbled back against the wall, only to see Dicko, firmly astride Jasper, charge the stable door which sprang open, releasing the flying duo onto the yard.

I recovered quickly and followed them out to witness one of the finest Bucking Boar Exhibitions one could wish to see, as Dicko, raving like a dervish and still brandishing the boot and jug, rode Jasper around the yard.

Eventually, after about five circuits, they parted company and Dicko was deposited in a patch of docks by the water trough.

I stood, trying to contain my mirth, as Dicko scrambled to his feet.

'Rope snapped!' I said, holding up the frayed end. 'Sorry!'

'You looks as sorry as 'e does,' commented Dicko grumpily as he picked up his cap and looked at Jasper. The old boar seemed perfectly recovered and was tucking into the potato clamp with great energy.

'He's eating now,' I said, just suppressing a smile.

'Told yer it would work, didn't' I?' said Dicko, dusting down his moleskins.

Then, he gave one of his famous winks and said, 'Where's me flamin' bottle?' And we both burst out laughing.

During that summer Dicko taught me how to turn a sheep, tack up a cart horse, mix feed, tell good corn from bad, know when a cow was 'slacking' to calve or spot a beast not 'doing'. He taught me how to observe with a countryman's eye and follow the signs of nature.

There was one point of observation for which I shall particularly remember Dicko. We had been slaving all morning to dig a post-hole for the gateway leading from the cow pasture onto the canal lane. From the spot where we were working the land fell away gently, presenting a superb view of the countryside, right down to the river several miles away. Dicko, bare to the waist, his torso glistening with sweat, was resting with his weight on his shovel, when down the lane came a smartly dressed young man with a giggling little blonde on his arm.

Dicko touched his cap and said, 'Goodmorning.'

'Digging a hole for that post, eh!' commented the young gentleman, rather snootily.

Dicko nodded.

The young man stepped gingerly forward and peered over the edge.

'Not quite deep enough,' he said, after some consideration.

Dicko straightened up on his shovel and I tensed, wondering what was coming next.

'An 'ow would you be knowin' that, then?' asked Dicko, slowly.

'I could be wrong,' replied the young man, with a cocky smile. 'I'm only a civil engineer, but I'm pretty sure that hole is too shallow.'

'Come along, darling,' said the girl. 'Don't stop the men working.' Then she gave a little gasp. 'Oh, look!' she said, suddenly. 'Down there. That cow — why hasn't it got any horns?'

The young man turned and looked in the direction she was pointing: to an animal grazing near the larch wood, two fields away.

'I say, my dear chap,' he said, turning to Dicko, who was still leaning on his shovel. 'You can see it. Tell me, why hasn't that cow got any horns?'

I was just about to blurt out a comment, when Dicko caught my eye.

'Well, sir,' he began, slowly, 'there be many reasons why cows don't 'ave horns. Some cows is born without 'em. Some cows gets 'em knocked off. And with some cows, we cuts 'em off. But that animal down there ain't got horns for a different reason.'

'Oh,' said the young man. 'Tell me, now. Why is that?'

'Well, sir, I may be wrong,' said Dicko, leaning forward and lowering his tone rather confidentially. 'I'm only a country bloke, but I'm pretty sure that cow down there is a 'orse!'

That summer at Brynheulog was one of the happiest of my life and, although the prospect of returning to the fog and grime of a Glasgow winter was daunting, my appetite for a country life had been well and truly whetted.

*   *   *

Back in Glasgow, I changed my digs and went to live in a small 'semi' in Anniesland, which I shared with a pal of mine. Our landlady and her longsuffering husband had been in service to some gentry in Argyll and had returned to the city to retire. Mrs Maddox treated Jack and me like gentry too, even though we could afford little and her budget was slim. But she was kindness itself, and often when we came in from our studies, cold and wet, she would make us a tonic she called 'Bosun's Cream'. It looked not unlike Dicko's jollop and consisted of milk, whisky, some spice and a raw egg. Mrs Maddox would stand over us, until we, not wishing to offend her by refusing, had consumed the slimy beverage.

'Do you'se like it?' she would ask, topping up our glasses. I would nod and say it was very good, adding, 'It's Jack's favourite.' And Jack, who could only just keep the concoction down, would give me hell when we got up to our room.

Mrs Maddox was a diminutive lady, neat as a new pin and with a heart of gold, but she had one slight weakness: she loved a 'wee flutter'.

Twice a week found her at the greyhound track, all on her own, amongst the roughs and toughs of the city, and nearly always she came back with the same tale.

'There I was,' she would begin, as she took off her hat and carefully removed the long spiky pin. 'There I was, marking my card. An' I thought I'd do three and two and four and seven reversed, when this man came and stood in front of me. "What are you'se doing?" asked I. "Five and three and one and six reversed, dearie," says he. He seemed ever so nice, so I changed — and what do you'se think?' Mrs Maddox would stand, her coat half off, waiting for our response which invariably came in unison.

'Three and two and four and seven reversed, came up!'

'Ay, it did!' she would say, shaking her head. 'I should never have listened to that useless fellow.' Completely forgetting that it was her fault for being nosey.

Occasionally she got it right and would be beaming like a little sun when she arrived home. But she rarely brought her winnings, for she would have spent them at the shops where she would buy a chicken for the following day's dinner.

'A wee treat,' she would say.

Which is probably another reason why I shall always regard roast chicken as something rather special.

Part of the Autumn term was spent under the tuition of the great Professor Bardsley, known affectionately as the Bomber, for if one was unfortunate enough to incur his displeasure he was apt to come down on his victim swiftly and from a great height, with devastating effect.

At his first lecture he stood before us, dressed sombrely but immaculately in a black suit with tie to match, his shoes sparkling in the lecture room lights. His most distinguishing feature was a mat of heavily greased black hair, topping a sallow complexion and hooked nose that combined to give him the appearance of an up-market funeral director — which was quite apt, considering his subject.

'Pathology!' he boomed. 'From the Greek! *Pathos* — suffering! *Logos* — discourse!'

Then he lowered his tone and, in the manner of Talfyn Thomas, Chief Warden of Abergranog, hissed:

'Gentlemen, I am going to teach you about suffering!'

I never forgot it.

But the learned Professor led us through the pathways

of death and decay carefully and with dignity. He taught that disease and degeneration were not to be regarded as terrible enemies, but part of life's natural pattern of reaction and response. With this understanding, the clinician was more able to control the conditions and appreciate that, ultimately, even death was part of the orderly but irrevocable process.

But when the Professor did adopt his 'Bomber' tactics, he could reduce anyone by verbal barrage to a heap of dust. For me, his most memorable tirade, after questioning a poor student who never seemed to get anything right, came when in exasperation the Bomber threw up his arms and roared: 'A million sperms and one of them had to be you!'

But if Pathology was a 'dead' subject, Materia Medica was quite lively fun. Due to some staffing problems at the college, we commenced the subject with lectures given by a temporary tutor, a jovial little Irishman who astounded us on the first day with his opening remarks:

'Materia Medica used to be a lot of balls!'

He grinned mischievously and, having seen that his comment had achieved the desired effect, qualified it by saying: 'Horse balls, of course. Balls for coughs. Balls for water. Balls for blood. Balls to stop and balls to start — like I said . . .' he peered over the top of his half-rimmed spectacles in anticipation of the inevitable chorus that dutifully arose from the class:

'JUST A LOT OF BALLS!'

In fact, the 1950s were seeing a tremendous change in human and animal therapy, with the advent of antibiotics and drugs in injectable form. We were probably some of the last students to learn the practicalities of pharmacy and were taught how to make pills, pack powders and prepare medicines from ingredients whose names suggested hidden powers and mysterious potency: Kamala, Male Fern, Croton Oil and Sweet Spirit of Nitre.

When the drench or the draught was prepared, each one could be tailor-made for the patient, with a bit of this and a touch of that, all mixed freshly and presented, corked and labelled, in a great glass bottle. Far more impressive than a few millilitres of colourless liquid quickly injected under the skin.

The instructions for administration were also far more picturesque. 'A wineglassful to be given in a pint of old ale, morning and night.' 'Mix thoroughly in a pint of gruel' or 'Dilute with a quart of spring water.'

We were being taught the art and science of veterinary medicine and I think that in the presentation of their treatments, the old veterinarians extolled the art to the full.

Another subject I found most fascinating was the study of parasites — worms, flukes, ticks, fleas and countless minute beings that, by their natural ingenuity, were able to exist, feed and reproduce by courtesy of some unsuspecting animal body. Of course, they contributed nothing towards the well-being of their hosts, and the damage they created caused loss of condition and even death as a result, but still, the complexity of their existence could not be discarded lightly.

There were so many uninvited guests in the animal world — the horse bots that could live quite happily in the stomach without themselves being digested, or the warble fly whose larva burrowed through the skin on a cow's hoof and migrated through the tissues until it reached the back, where it rested through the winter, breathing through a small hole which it made between the hairs.

While the parasites may have been insignificant in appearance, many of them rejoiced in names of such grandeur that in some cases they defied pronunciation. There was a minute stomach worm of the horse, four millimetres long, called *Paranplocephala mamillana*, its name longer than its body. A midge, only a millimetre bigger, known as *Phlebotomus papatasii*. And it's quite amazing how some of these names, despite their complexity, can hang on in the memory. There was a small mite found only in Japan, called *Trombicula akamushi*, that was responsible for a disease called Tsutsugamushi Disease — why I remember it, I do not know and whether this obscure fact will ever be any use to me is doubtful, to say the least. But the student mind functions in weird and wonderful ways and mine was no exception.

*   *   *

By now, the grounding that we had been given over the previous three years was beginning to gel, so that the structure and function of animals, bacteria and parasites, and their inter-relationships, were becoming clearer. The effects of the available medicines and the value of correct diets had been investigated, but still we had not been let loose on real live animals and indeed, before we were, there was one other important part of the veterinary education that had to be undertaken.

Seeing animals in specially designed veterinary teaching hospitals is an admirable way of demonstrating how disease should be diagnosed and prevented or treated. But applying the art and science of veterinary medicine under more natural conditions, such as windswept fields, dimly lit barns, kitchen tables or small surgeries, can be vastly different. In order, therefore, to obtain the correct balance, the vacations now had to be spent with a veterinary surgeon in what is termed 'Seeing Practice'.

It was my extreme good fortune to be taken as a student by Christopher John Pink, MRCVS, who practised from his residence at Barrow Hill in Newpool, about twelve miles from Abergranog.

Christopher John Pink, or C.J. as he was more commonly known, was a bustling, jovial Welshman, grey-haired and balding, with a bushy moustache that stretched an extra two inches whenever he smiled.

In his fifties, C.J. always dressed in the manner of a country squire, even though not all his clients were on the estates and large farms of the Usk valley. His practice extended well up into the mining valleys, where at the windswept hill farms and smallholdings, he was a great favourite and highly respected.

Immaculate, in sharp-fitting cavalry twill trousers and three-quarter length hacking jacket in a loud check, he was always on the move. The only feature that detracted from his complete sartorial elegance was the fact that, whatever he picked up, in the nature of small bottles, bits of bandage, pencils, string or messages on pieces of paper, he stuffed into his jacket pockets so that they bulged like saddlebags.

Occasionally, when his wife cornered him and demanded he sort them out, he would empty the contents onto the surgery table and, after reforming them in small matching piles, put three-quarters of them back into his pockets.

'You're a proper jackdaw,' Mrs Pink would say, shaking her head. At which remark, C.J. would flap his elbows at his sides like wings and kiss her on the cheek. 'And that's a quick peck,' he'd say, with a cheeky grin, his moustache lengthening considerably.

Another distinctive feature of that warmhearted Welshman was the way he would rub his hands together, gleefully, as if constantly excited by the prospect of whatever was to come. And indeed he was, for C.J. enjoyed his veterinary work to the full and had a wealth of practical experience to offer. Much of his sound advice was contained in what he termed 'Pink's Law', the quoting of which was always accompanied by the raising of the right index finger, as if to call attention, followed by a gentle tapping of the nose with the same finger and a closing of the left eye.

'Communication is the key to success,' he would expound, finger raised. Then the tapping and the closed eye. 'Whether it be man or animal!'

And C.J. was an artist in communication, treating all his clients with an equivalent degree of respect and good humour, such that in his company they relaxed and were completely confident in his expertise, whether it was Widow Evans and her mangy mongrel or Lord Bogan and his hunter.

But it was with animals that the man was in a class on his own, and though, during my future years, I was to see many vets in action, there was none to equal him in communicating with his patients.

'Talk, touch and treat them as an equal,' he told me, when I asked his secret. 'They, too, have feelings, and they're far more honest and direct about showing them.'

When he handled animals, C.J. was gentle but firm. He talked and touched, but as he did so he was all the time observing and examining. This latter feature may well have escaped the notice of the casual onlooker, for one couldn't help but believe, by his attitude, that the animal understood his every word.

'Now m'dear,' he'd say in a comforting tone to a fat old Friesian cow overdue with the birth of her calf. 'You'll be glad to get this load off your mind, no doubt.' Then, he'd commence his examination, chatting away all the time to her, until finally he would say: 'Nothing to worry about. Just keep your strength up and in a few days it will all be over.'

Or there was the time he reprimanded a battle-scarred tom cat, as a doctor might his company director patient. 'Slow it down a bit,' he said, wagging his finger at the dishevelled creature, who hung it's tattered head in disgrace. 'If you don't, you'll pop off before your time.'

But the classic example of C.J.'s art of communication was, for me, an experience I shall never forget.

It concerned a dog called Prince.

'We're going to see Mrs Webster, the landlady at the Black Lion,' announced C.J., one morning. 'You'll be interested in this case, it's what you might call an excercise in communication. How well can you sing?'

A little taken aback by his question, I smiled and shook my head.

'Do you know "Sospan Fach"?' he asked, grinning.

'The first verse, but what's that got to do with it?'

'Communication,' said C.J. 'That's what it's all about.'

With a chuckle he pressed the starter and the old Vauxhall rattled into life. As we set off down into Newpool, he explained.

'Mrs Webster's got a dog called Prince. An Alsatian, quite old, partly blind and not very sociable. But since her husband died three years ago, he's helped her keep the pub in order; the Black Lion's down near the Dock and the clientele can get a bit rough.' We stopped at the lights and the engine cut out. C.J. cursed softly and pressed the starter.

'When I first went to see him, shortly after she'd been widowed, I couldn't get near the old rascal. Quite vicious he was. I was a little worried about giving him a sedative because of his age and was wondering what I should do, when Mrs Webster said, "Try singing." Apparently Alf, her husband, used to sing to old Prince a lot and, according to Mrs Webster, the old dog would lie down and let Alf do what he liked with him.' C.J. slammed on the brakes as a cyclist cut across the junction in front of us and cursed again.

'What did you sing?' I asked.

'Well,' he continued, 'she said Alf sang Rugby songs, but I didn't think I could sing some of the ones I knew in front of Mrs Webster, so I tried "Sospan Fach".'

'And it worked?' I asked.

'Like a charm, boy. Must have hit the jackpot first time. The old dog stopped barking and lay down on the mat and I was able to treat him. He was suffering from bad ears and he let me clean and dress them, no bother at all.'

'What's the trouble this time?'

'A bad paw. Won't let anyone touch it. All I hope is, he's still in a musical frame of mind.'

C.J. swung the Vauxhall into a rather dingy street lined with terraced houses; at the far end the derricks of the dockyard and assorted funnels of berthed coasters blocked out the skyline. Halfway down the street we pulled up outside the Black Lion.

The pub was no more than a double-fronted terraced

house that had been painted with a heavy coat of black paint or pitch, giving it a rather sinister appearance.

I followed C.J. through the half-open door into the bar; the sharp tang of scented smoke cut the back of my throat and made my eyes water slightly. There were several men of mixed nationality drinking, who took no notice of us until a blonde woman behind the bar called out:

'Thank's for coming, Mr Pink. He's in the kitchen. Can you manage, I'm a bit busy for the moment?'

'Leave it to us,' said C.J.

Then the blonde woman caught sight of me.

'Does the young man know about Prince?' she asked, slightly nervously.

'Yes,' said C.J. 'Champion tenor from Abergranog. He'll have old Prince eating out of his hand.'

'Or eatin' 'is 'and!' said one of the men leaning on the bar. 'Rather 'ew than me, boyo.'

I followed C.J. up a narrow passage beside the bar to a small hallway in which were three doors. He pointed to one, set down his bag and began to whisper.

'When we start singing he'll bark like hell. But as long as we don't stop he's all right. You take the bag and if I want anything, I'll sing it to you. He doesn't mind what the words are so long as you keep up the tune.'

He must have seen the perplexed look on my face, because he added: 'Don't worry, boy. Not all my patients are like this. Now one, two, three . . .'

And with that, he placed his hand on the door knob and burst into song.

Instantly our singing triggered off a ferocious barking from behind the door. It sounded more like a pack of wolves, and when he opened the door I could see why.

Prince was big, black and mean. 'Fang' should have been his name, for his gaping jaws showed a set of dentures that would have done a tiger proud.

C.J. waved his palm upwards to indicate that increased volume was desirable, his rich tenor voice fighting against the savage barking.

It was at that point that my mouth went dry, possibly from the smoke of the bar — or I forgot the words — or I was frightened.

C.J. waved his hand more vigorously.

My voice came back and I sang out loud.

Prince came towards me, not casually, but with intention. C.J. waved his hand, and sang 'Sospan Fach' for all he was worth.

> 'I think we've got him where we want him,
> He likes you, keep singing the same tune.
> I'm sure that he'll lie down in a minute,
> Just move the bag and let me have more room.'

As I picked up the medical bag, Prince turned away from me and, after taking a look at the kitchen mat, made a wide circle, yawned and lay down full length.

To the tune of 'Sospan Fach', C.J. gave me further instructions.

> 'Look now, the right paw is quite swollen,
> I'll search it and see what I can find.
> Just keep an eye upon his head, now,
> In case he goes for my behind.'

But Prince had been lulled into a trance; 'Sospan Fach' had done the trick. And as I stood in the Black Lion kitchen, medical bag in hand, watching C.J. tending to Prince and singing softly as he did so, I wondered if Glasgow University had ever considered singing an essential part of the veterinary curriculum.

Still crooning, C.J. continued to examine Prince's pad. Suddenly he plucked his hand backwards, and between his fingers I saw a small sliver of wood.

> 'This is the cause of all the trouble,
> Splinter from the boards upon the floor.
> In the case you'll find a tube of ointment
> And I'll put some on the septic sore.'

Still adding to the chorus, I opened the case and took out

the ointment. C.J. dressed Prince's pad and when he'd finished, stood up and sang:

> 'Right, Hugh, now I think we've finished,
> Dressed it, I can't do any more.
> You're doing very well now, just keep singing,
> Then gently back out through the door.'

Prince still lay stretched out upon the mat as C.J. eased away from him and drew back through the door behind me.

'Communication,' he said, as he turned the knob. 'You can stop singing now, boy. Come on, I'll buy you a pint.'

On the way back to the surgery, I lay back in the seat, shattered by the experience.

'Reminded me a bit of Androcles and the lion,' I said.

'Funny you should mention him,' said C.J., wrestling with the windscreen wiper knob, for it had now started raining. 'Always thought he must have had a bit of a trick going for him.'

'Probably had some Welsh blood,' I suggested.

'Wonder what he was singing,' said C.J. peering through the half cleaned screen.

'"Onward Christian Soldiers",' I said.

'Bound to be,' said C.J., slapping the wheel. 'I might even try that next time.'

But I never knew whether he did.

The veterinary surgeons of C.J.'s era were certainly not motivated by financial gain. 'Veterinary surgery is a way of life and not a job,' he would say. And for him, that was not a Law, but a belief — and so it had to be, for both animals and clients showed no concern for time or place and often the nights were as busy as the days.

Only rarely did he show the strain. One of the few occasions was a Sunday night, just on eight o'clock, when, after a particularly hectic day the phone bell tinkled once again.

C.J. wearily lifted up the instrument and took the call.

After several minutes of conversation, during which time his only contribution was to say 'Yes' about six times, he eventually answered, 'As soon as we can!' and banged the receiver down.

He covered his face with his hand, drawing it downwards, as if trying to wipe away his tiredness.

'Elmer Morgan, Ty-Bran,' he said, finally. 'Hill farmer, bachelor, Baptist and skinflint, has a cow calving.' He stood up, put his hands on his hips and bent his body backwards. 'Been calving since daybreak, look you,' he continued, with an exaggerated Welsh accent which I assumed was in the manner of Elmer Morgan. 'And now, Elmer, bless his tight old pockets, wants some help immediately — and if not, sooner!'

'Ty-Bran,' I said. 'That's Nantygyll way, isn't it?'

'Go through Nantygyll and up the mountain until you think you're in Heaven,' explained C.J. 'Then you're about half way there. Although on a night like this it will be more like the Other Place!'

'Bit late calling,' I commented.

'Been to Chapel, look you,' he replied. 'Twice every Sunday. Pity he isn't so regular about paying his bills — owes me for twelve months. Prays on his knees on a Sunday and on everyone else during the week.' Then C.J. rubbed his hands vigorously. 'Come on,' he said. 'None shall sleep.'

I smiled at his resilience and admired it too, for I knew he was very tired.

'Do you know that one?' he asked. 'It's from *Turandot* by Giacomo Puccini. I heard it at Covent Garden, in my twenties — pure magic!' And with that, he launched into the aria with great gusto and led off to the car.

It was nearly dark and spitting with rain as we drove through the narrow, shiny streets of the valley to Nantygyll. Once away from the monotonous rows of terraced houses that made up the small township, we took the mountain road where the track became rougher and more tortuous.

The windscreen wipers wing-wanged away with a force and noise that suggested a determined effort on their part; alas, the result was but a scrawling disturbance of the wet screen, for they were well past their best.

'Skin a flea for sixpence, then ask for expenses,' said C.J., as he peered into the driving rain. 'Twelve months overdue and calls me out on a filthy night like this. Who'd be a vet?'

'I would,' I replied.

He gave me a sideways glance, then he returned his gaze to the windscreen. A minute later he looked sideways again, this time he winked and grinned, so that his moustache extended a good two inches.

'Good,' he said cheerily. 'I'm glad of that. Let's go and sort out Elmer!'

With that he spurted the old Vauxhall forward and we rattled on up the track.

When we drove into the yard, Elmer was standing waiting for us in the rain — and just as C.J. had described him, so did he look.

Wind-blown, weathered, tall and slightly stooping, he had the appearance of a vulture. Over his shoulders he wore a corn sack, knotted at his chest, and around his waist, tied with string, was another one. A tall black hat topped his head and from the brim of it, thin streams of water ran down at intervals onto the saturated corn sack. Below the hat was the meanest face I had ever seen.

The Vauxhall squelched to a halt alongside and C.J. opened the window.

'Took 'ewer time, didn' 'ew!' squeaked Elmer sarcastically. Then he peered deeper into the car and his beady eye settled upon me. He raised a thin finger and poked it forward. 'Who's that?' he questioned.

'Hugh Lasgarn,' replied C.J.

'Student?' asked Elmer, suspiciously. 'Don' want no one learning on my cows. Too valuable, they are!'

'Hugh is my assistant,' retorted C.J. firmly. 'Where is

she?'

'On the bank,' he replied, shaking a small torrent from his hat.

'You could have got her in on a night like this,' said C.J. sharply.

'More natural out of doors,' said Elmer, equally sharply. 'Anyway, she's down.'

In the darkness of the car I contemplated the banter between farmer and vet. Elmer seemed to resent having to call C.J. for help — yet he needed him, or at least, his cow did. C.J., in turn, had responded to the call, on a filthy night, and a Sunday. He still had not been paid for his previous services over twelve months, but despite that was expected to co-operate. 'Who'd be a vet?' I asked myself, just as C.J. had, only minutes ago.

'Calving bag, ropes and medical case,' shouted C.J. as we emerged. 'What about water, Elmer?'

'Isn't this enough for 'ew?' Elmer Morgan lifted skywards the tilly lamp he was holding, illuminating shafts of Welsh Mountain rain, to which there is no equal for its wetting capacity. For a moment a suggestion of a smile crossed his sallow face, then his features froze again and he lowered the lamp.

'Took some up in a churn before 'ew come,' he said. 'Come back from Chapel, went up to look at 'er. Come back. Rang 'ew. Then took the water up.' He raised his lamp over the car as we changed into our boots and waterproofs. 'Knew I'd 'ave plenty of time,' he added.

But C.J. and I took no notice of his jibe; instead we checked our gear and, like all good vets, or nearly vets — kept our thoughts to ourselves.

In single file we left the yard through the mountain gate, the rain slashing against us. Elmer led with the tilly, I followed with calving bag and ropes and C.J. puffed away behind with the medical case.

On the ridge we rested.

'She is due now, is she?' asked C.J., in between gasps.

'Should have calved this morning,' said Elmer, setting

down the tilly, his voice clear and his breathing steady and unstressed — the benefit of a lifetime of hill farming. 'Looked on 'er at dawn, then again before I went to Chapel. Saw 'er when I come back and before I went again. To Chapel, 'ew see.' He shone the lamp and looked at us as if we had never heard of it. 'Then I went again, tonight.' Elmer Morgan hung his head as if he was apologising for what he was about to say next. 'When I came back, she was still the same — so I had to ring for 'ew.'

C.J. wiped the rain from his moustache and grinned.

'The Lord works in mysterious ways, Elmer,' he said, having regained his breath.

'Take not His name in vain, Mr Pink,' came the reply, but it was faceless, for Elmer had already turned and was leading off up the bank.

As we pushed on, the rain eased, and by the time we reached the small plateau at the top of the rise, I could see the lights of Nantygyll twinkling in the valley. In the distance came a grunting sound and soon the outline of a cow appeared, lying on the edge of the plateau. Even in the dark I could see her shape, and when Elmer raised his lamp I could see she was black.

Just like Old Thundertits.

C.J. set down his case and took a torch from his waterproof pocket. He walked round to the cow's head and shone the light. Again like Old Thundertits, her horns had dug into the soil and squirts of steam came from her nostrils and, apart from the fact that she was soaking wet, like the rest of us, it was Little Pant all over again.

'What's her name?' asked C.J., bending down.

'Megan,' said Elmer, irritably.

C.J. parted the old cow's eyelids gently. To some it might have appeared as if he was soothing and caressing the poor beast, but I knew he was starting his clinical examination and, as he talked, he was assessing the situation.

'You've picked a grand night to do this, Megan. Sunday's the Day of Rest, didn't you know?' He shone his torch over her flanks, then took out his stethoscope and listened to her heart.

'Calving she is,' Elmer informed C.J., rather impatiently.

C.J. paid no attention to the remark, but continued his examination. Finally, he shone his torch on the tailhead and pressed the ligaments beneath.

'She is ready to calve,' he said, addressing his comments to me. 'But something is definitely wrong. She's as dry as a bone behind and by now there should be some sign of the water.' He undid his waterproof and laid it on the grass, then he took off his jacket and shirt. Stripped to the waist in the gentle drizzle that now descended, he rolled his clothes in the waterproof and, donning his apron, turned to Elmer.

'Soap!'

Elmer ferreted beneath the sack around his waist, obviously searching for a pocket. Eventually he withdrew a piece of newspaper which he carefully unrolled — to reveal a scrap of soap about the size of a matchbox which, by its sharp edges, had no doubt been sliced from a larger bar.

'If cleanliness is next to godliness, you've got a long way to go, Elmer,' said C.J. Then working hard with the morsel, he soaped his arm up to his shoulder.

There are many ways of spending a Sunday night, even in Wales, and I remember thinking, as I held Megan's tail, while mean old Elmer shone the lamp and C.J., stripped to the waist, eased a soapy arm into the depths of the sweating, prostrate cow on the side of Nantygyll Mountain in the rain, that this must definitely be one of the more unusual.

As C.J. cautiously probed the birth canal, Megan began to strain uneasily.

'Pinch her back!' he called to Elmer.

Elmer, without any comment, set down the lamp and squeezed Megan's spine with his thin, scrawny hands.

'Further forward!' shouted C.J.

Elmer moved to her shoulders and his lean frame tensed as he squeezed again.

'Stops the muscle contractions and eases the straining,' said C.J., looking up at me, and as he did so I could see the tension in his rain-spattered face.

'Feel anything?' enquired Elmer urgently, still bent and squeezing. C.J. didn't answer, but gradually withdrew his arm, sat back on his haunches and sighed.

'What is it, mun?' shrieked Elmer. 'For God's sake, what is it?'

C.J. rose to his feet. 'Elmer Morgan,' he said, 'don't blaspheme. We are going to need all the help available. You. Hugh. Megan, who's already doing her best.' C.J. looked upwards into the murky gloom. 'And Anyone Else who might care to lend a hand!' he added, wiping the rain from his face.

'What is it? What is it?' Elmer shone the lamp right in C.J.'s face.

'It's a twisted womb,' he said.

And I realised then, that it wasn't like Old Thundertits after all.

Elmer Morgan covered his face with his hand. 'Megan, my best cow,' he wailed. 'My best cow.'

'I must say that one bit of Providence is that you didn't get her in to the cowhouse, Elmer,' remarked C.J. as he opened the calving bag and uncoiled a length of rope. 'The fact that we're on the hill will make it easier to roll her. And I want Hugh to feel it, too,' he added, firmly, 'so that he will know which way I want the rope to be pulled.'

Elmer made no comment and C.J. nodded to me to make an internal examination. I quickly stripped, soaped my arm with the morsel of soap and knelt down behind Megan. C.J. knelt alongside and, as I gently inserted my hand, he explained what I would feel.

'If she strains, don't force against it. Wait until she relaxes, then smoothly ease in.'

I had felt normal calvings on two previous occasions, so the sensation was not completely unknown to me.

'Let your hand go with the contour and you'll find the passage twisted like a corkscrew. Feel it?'

The tissue was warm and tacky, but in no way objectionable. In fact, now that I was directly involved, my mind was just concentrating on what I could discover by touch.

'Yes,' I replied, as my arm started to twist naturally with the folds of tissue.

'Now,' said C.J. 'I want you to do something which every vet must learn to do, and learn to do well. I want you to see with your fingers.'

When he said it, 'See with your fingers', I nearly said, 'that's just what I'm doing.' For I realised that, while I was on my knees gazing into the darkness of the night, in my mind was a picture of the convoluted channel which was preventing the calf's delivery.

'Which way is it going?' asked C.J. 'Clockwise or anti-clockwise?'

I felt the side of the channel, one way, then the other. Although my mental picture seemed quite clear, I couldn't decide.

'Confusing, isn't it?' he said. 'Come out carefully and I'll show you how to check. Elmer, give me that sack from around your waist.'

Without a murmur, Elmer untied the sack and handed it over, and as C.J. explained the circumstances to me, the old farmer listened intently.

'As you know, Hugh,' he began, 'for the calf inside the womb, it's rather like being in a water-filled balloon. In the early stages it lies in a crouched position, but in the later stages, shortly before birth, it extends into a sort of diving posture, head between legs, which are pointed towards the neck of the womb. Imagine this sack as the womb and this as the neck, called the cervix.'

C.J. held up the sack by its far corner, then gathered up the open end in his other hand. 'That's the normal position. When the neck opens, out comes the calf.' He relaxed his grip on the neck of the sack. 'Now, in Megan's case, unfortunately, the calf in extending has caused the womb to rotate — so!' He twisted the neck of the sack and held it up. 'Look at this!' He held the gathered end towards me. 'Which way are the folds?'

'Anticlockwise!' Both Elmer and I answered in unison.

'Correct!' C.J. gave the neck of the sack a further twist to confirm our answer. 'Now. To undo it we have to turn Megan in the same direction, but keep the womb still, so that she can catch up upon the twist. See?'

'How d'yew reckon to do that, then?' said Elmer, more in despair than sarcasm. 'Yew'm on Nantygyll Mountain now, mind. Not Porthcawl Fairground!'

'I shall put my arm into the neck of the womb and hold it as steady as I can,' explained C.J., holding up the rope from the calving bag. 'We'll tie this to Megan's feet, then you and Hugh stand below her, down the slope, and when I give the word you jerk her right over. It must be quick, so that her body turns faster than the womb, which I will attempt to slow down.'

'Deu, man,' said Elmer. 'Sounds a performance.'

'Just hold this and stop your rattle,' said C.J. 'You'll need all your wind to pull!' With that, he made double nooses in the rope ends and attached them to Megan's underside fore and hind legs. Then, washing up again, he knelt down behind the cow and gave the final instructions.

'D'yew think the calf is alive?' asked Elmer, as he spat on his hands in readiness for the rope.

'If you said the right words in Chapel, there's a good chance,' came the reply.

'Mr Pink!' rasped Elmer, then he took up the strain.

'When I say "now",' said C.J., 'and not before. But make it strong and quick.'

He lay flat out this time, on the sodden mountain turf, legs splayed to give himself more stability. Then he eased his arm inside Megan as Elmer and I pulled the rope taut.

Megan gave a heave as C.J. took up his position. He let her relax and, as she did, shouted:

'PULL!'

Elmer and I jerked backwards and heaved. Megan rose

onto her back and I heard C.J. gasp as he held firm. Then my foot slipped on the grass and I lost my grasp and Megan rolled back on her side.

'Sorry,' I said.

'We'll try again,' said Elmer, gruffly. He gave a great sniff, spat on his hands and took fresh hold of the rope.

With renewed effort we pulled again at C.J.'s command. This time, Megan rose onto her back and a further quick jerk forced her to flop right over onto her other side.

'Any good, man?' Elmer's voice echoed over the hillside as he shouted.

C.J. lay still and exhausted for a few seconds, then, with a sigh he said: 'Not quite.'

It took two more rolls, leaving us a good ten yards down the hill, before he eventually shouted: 'Enough!' And indeed, it was enough, for in seconds the waters, now released, came gushing out and in five minutes, with a little assistance, a fine Friesian cross Hereford calf slithered into the world on Nantygyll Mountain that Sunday night.

Everyone, including Megan, breathed a sigh of relief.

'Is it all right?' Elmer shone the tilly over the glistening, writhing body. The calf bawled, a watery choking sound.

'Pick it up by its back legs,' shouted C.J., 'and jerk it!'

I grabbed the right and Elmer the left; it was slippery and heavy, but we raised it together.

'Up and down,' C.J. waved his hands. 'Probably got some fluid in its throat; that will shake it out.' And sure enough, as we shook, the calf coughed and started to breathe more easily. We laid it on the ground and Elmer picked up the lamp again.

'What do you think of that, then?' asked C.J., washing his bespattered torso with water from the churn.

Elmer held the tilly closer and lifted the calf's hind leg, then he grunted with disgust.

'A bull!' he said. 'An' I wanted a 'effer!'

C.J. stopped his ablutions and turned his back on us, looking down the bank to the twinkling lights of Nantygyll. I saw him breathe deeply, then he stood quite still for several minutes. Eventually he moved and confronted Megan, who by now was sitting up and looking much more cheerful.

'Did you hear that, Megan?' he said to the old cow. 'He wanted a heifer!' Then he put his hands on her forehead and added, 'Aren't there times when you feel like packing it all in?'

By the time we had collected up the gear, Megan was up and nuzzling her calf. The transformation from the immobile hulk she had been to a vigorous, tail-swishing mother was remarkable.

''Old the light while I try 'er tits,' said Elmer, handing me the lamp. Cautiously he leaned against the cow and his sinewy hands clasped each teat in turn and with a firm downward draw sent streams of first-milk onto the wet grass where it formed a small frothy pool.

'Plenty there — 'e'll be all right,' he commented, taking back the lamp. ''Ew can wash at the house an' I'll make 'ew some tea.'

'Right,' said C.J., slipping his waterproof loosely over his shoulders. 'A wash will be fine, but no tea, thanks.'

'As 'ew wish.' As Elmer led off, C.J. turned to me and whispered:

'Herbal tea. Aaach! Like gypsy's shaving water.' He held his finger to his lips, indicating that I should not pursue the subject.

The kitchen at Ty-Bran was a corrugated tin lean-to at the back of the whitewashed farmhouse. Damp, uneven flagstones covered the floor and, just inside the door, a shallow brown stone sink sat upon two low brick pillars. Above it, a dim unshaded light bulb weakly illuminated the interior. Elmer took a large kettle from an oil stove and poured the steaming contents into a bowl in the sink, and as the vapour rose it misted up a piece of cracked mirror glass fixed to the wall above. On a wooden shelf to one side stood a Victoria and Albert shaving mug out of which poked a shaving soap stick and a great hairy shaving brush; alongside the mug lay a cut-throat razor. My mind ran back to Mr Ellis' kitchen and Boggy, and I found my eyes roaming the walls — and sure enough they were there, on the far wall, hanging from a nail, just what I might have expected to be part of Elmer Morgan's lifestyle: a bunch of wicked, thin-wired snares. I watched him as he carefully cut another morsel of soap from a long narrow bar and decided that piety of Elmer Morgan's sort was no antidote to meanness and cruelty.

He ladled some cold water from a tin bath into the bowl and in turn we washed. The water was warm and soft and the soap lathered readily, but had a rather austere, disinfectant aroma that one associates with certain institutions. The towel was a bleached sack, bound at the edges with linen tape. Through a half open door leading from the lean-to, I glimpsed the living room which looked reasonably comfortable, with a bright fire burning in the tall, black-leaded iron grate. A table in the centre was cluttered with crockery and foodstuffs, while in the corner stood a grandfather clock with a faded, painted face.

C.J. reclothed himself after washing and, as he came to the last buttons of his shirt neck, turned to Elmer who was standing, silently, behind.

'Your account with me is outstanding by twelve months, Elmer,' he said, very directly. 'Thirty-nine pounds seven shillings and sixpence, to be exact — not counting tonight. It's about time you settled.'

'Yes, Mr Pink.' Elmer shuffled uncomfortably. 'I'll settle.'

'Settle the overdue now and you can leave tonight's on the book,' said C.J., reasonably.

'Settle now!' Elmer squeaked.

'Yes,' said C.J. 'Why not, man?'

Elmer stepped forward a pace, shoulders drooped, neck bent and beaky nose prominent, just like a vulture.

'Mr Pink,' he croaked, narrowing his beady eyes, 'you should know better than to ask.' Then he stood back, straightened, and held up his hand. 'It is the Sabbath!'

'The Sabbath!' exclaimed C.J., raising his bushy

eyebrows.

'I never do business with money on the Lord's day,' said Elmer, with fabricated reverence.

'I calved your cow for you on the Lord's day!' retorted C.J.

'Ministering to the sick,' said Elmer, slyly. 'That's what that is.'

C.J. grunted, then he leaned back upon his heels and glanced through the door into the living room.

'What's that clock say, Hugh?' He screwed up his eyes in an attempt to read the painted face.

'Eleven thirty,' I replied.

'Eleven thirty,' said C.J., smoothing down his moustache. 'Now there's a thing. What would you say to a cup of tea?'

I hesitated, remembering his whispered comment on the mountainside. Seeing my hesitation, he nodded his head towards me slowly.

'Oh. Yes,' I said. 'Thank you, Mr Morgan. That would be grand.'

C.J. turned upon Elmer, who had suddenly appeared to become smaller and meaner as he clasped his thin fingers together. In comparison C.J. exuded health and confidence and rubbed his strong, broad hands together warmly, as he did in anticipation of some pleasure to come.

'We'll take you up on your offer of tea, Elmer,' he said, smiling benevolently. 'And while you're making it, we'll have a warm by the fire. Then in half an hour or so, Hugh and I will be off!'

Then he stood back, bowed slightly, raised his hand and invited me to precede him into the living room.

It was getting on for half past twelve when we rattled off down the track in the old Vauxhall. The rain had stopped, leaving a dry, clear night, and as we reached the mountain gate, C.J. pulled up.

'Not a bad way to start the week, eh!' he said. 'Twisted

womb, live calf and we prised some cash out of Elmer, to boot.'

'I shall never forget the look on his face when you said we'd stop for half an hour or so,' I said.

'Neither shall I.' C.J. clapped his hands with delight. 'What did you think of the tea?'

'I've never tasted gypsy's shaving water, but that must be a fair description,' I agreed.

'But three cups a piece is a bit too much,' said C.J., flinging open the car door.

'You're right,' I said, getting out the other side.

And laughing heartily, we fired two streams of filtered herbal tea down the mountainside towards the twinkling lights of Nantygyll.

*   *   *

Christopher John Pink qualified at the Royal Veterinary College in 1924 and spent his first two years as an assistant in one of the largest horse practices in East London at that time.

C.J. must have made a most impressive sight as he drove his gig and high-stepper on his calls. Dressed immaculately in bowler hat, riding coat, breeches and leggings, with kid gloves and a silver stamped whip, he was very much the professional man.

'The ladies never stood a chance, boy,' he would say gleefully, when he talked of his early days. 'But you had to be sharp and stay sharp; there were as many amateur horse doctors and rogues about in those days as there were horses — and that was a lot. All ready to take a young vet for a ride, in more ways than one. Some of those fellows could really try your education, and examination of horses for soundness was a trial for horse and veterinary surgeon. There's many a way of leading a lame horse to make him look sound, or of settling his wind for a few hours. Thorough clinical examination was essential — and still is! Pink's Law: "Never make a spot diagnosis",' he added.

I remember showing some puzzlement when I first heard that remark.

'If it's got spots,' he explained, 'it could be a Dalmatian.' Then he tapped his nose gently with his forefinger and added, 'On the other hand, it could be a leopard!' C.J. rubbed his hands together. 'Always examine thoroughly and completely; never go on one factor alone, even if you are convinced you know the answer at first sight.' And that piece of advice was to prove invaluable on several occasions during my later career.

However, I did see C.J. hoisted by his own petard on one occasion, just at the end of his morning surgery, only about a week after he had imparted that particular section of Pink's Law to me.

It had been a busy surgery by Barrow Hill standards, with itchy dogs, lame cats, two budgerigars with overgrown beaks and a rabbit with a bad ear, when the last client walked through the door.

The contrast between owner and animal could not have been more complete, for while the former was a dishevelled, down-at-heel Irish tinker wrapped in wellworn, illfitting overcoat, tied with string, his charge was a handsome, brindle greyhound, sharp, alert and a picture of fitness.

'Cut 'is leg, so he did,' said the Irishman, scraping a tattered cap from his head and crumpling it up in his right hand. 'Bit o' bottle glass, sir, I think.'

'Been to a party, have you now?' said C.J., kneeling down and addressing the dog, who nuzzled sociably into his jacket pocket. 'What's your name?' he asked, stroking the elegant head, as if expecting the animal to reply.

''Tis Brown Arrow, sir,' the Irishman informed him.

'That's a posh name for a pal,' said C.J., still apparently talking to the dog. 'But he looks after you well, by the shine on you.'

'Oh, I do, sir, I do,' the Irishman confirmed enthusiastically. 'He's worth a lot to me, so he is, sir. An awful lot.'

'Good companions are hard to find,' said C.J., running

his hands over Brown Arrow's solid form. 'Let's have a look at this cut.' Then, with a smooth, swift motion he rose and lifted the dog and gently placed him on the examination table.

''Tis that one, there.' The Irishman pointed to the right foreleg.

C.J. raised the limb to reveal a skin lesion of about an inch, just above the outer pad. Before he passed any comment, he gave Brown Arrow a quick general examination, just in case he had missed anything — Pink's Law in practice.

'Nasty little gash,' he commented finally, 'but a couple of stitches should soon put the job right. Don't worry, old fellow,' he said, turning to the Irishman. 'We'll soon have your pal as right as rain.'

Out of the client's ear-shot, I helped C.J. get the instruments and suture materials together.

'Get a few of these tinker boyos in from time to time,' said C.J. quietly. 'Not bad old chaps, in the main. On the road usually, with just a dog for a companion. Poor but happy and think the world of their animals.'

'Brown Arrow looks in good condition,' I commented.

'Probably goes without, himself, to feed it,' said C.J., selecting a fine curved needle from his box.

'Fancy name, though,' I said. 'Just for a pet.'

'These boyos are romantics at heart,' replied C.J., drawing the local anaesthetic into a syringe. 'Come on, let's start the embroidery.'

Brown Arrow never flinched when the fine needle was inserted and the local spread around. C.J. expertly drew the wound edges together in fine, delicate sutures. Following a light dressing, the wound was bandaged and a small injection of penicillin given to ward off any infection.

'Should heal in about seven days,' he informed the Irishman, as he lifted the greyhound down from the table. 'And I've put in sutures that will dissolve, so there will be no problem about taking them out.'

'Appreciate it, I do, sir. Oh, indeed I do,' said the

Irishman, grabbing C.J.'s hand and shaking it vigorously. 'That dog, sir, is worth a lot to me.'

'I'm sure he is,' said C.J. smiling benevolently. 'I'm sure he is.'

'Now, what would you want me to be paying you, sir?' asked the Irishman.

'Oh, a pound to you. Just to cover the drugs,' C.J. replied, putting a hand on the old fellow's shoulder.

'Are ye sure, now?' he replied, eyebrows raised.

'If that's all right,' said C.J.

'Sure an it is,' said the Irishman, and with that he delved deeply into his greatcoat pocket and his hand emerged with a massive wad of notes.

It was the most money I had ever seen in one lump and it must have been the same for C.J., for he gasped, fell back a little and had to put his hand behind him onto the examination table to steady himself.

'Where did you get all that?' he asked, when he had recovered from the shock.

'Last night's winnings at Pontyglyn track with me auld dog, sir,' said the Irishman, gently waving the wad up and down and momentarily hypnotising C.J. 'Third time we've cleaned up in Wales this month, sir. Told yer he was worth a lot to me, an' so he is. Offered five hundred pounds for him only last night, so I was, but if I hang out I reckon I'll get twice of that afore I'm finished.' Then, with a great flourish, he peeled a pound note from the top of the pile. 'Now there is your fee, sir, an' a gen'lman ye are too.' Then he peeled off another pound. 'And I'd like you an' your young man here to have a drink on me an' Brown Arrow, for all yer kindness, sir, so I would.'

He placed the two notes in C.J.'s limp hand and, pushing his cap untidily back onto his balding head, bid us both 'Goodmornin'.

When he had gone, C.J. shut the door behind him and leaned heavily against it.

'A pound,' he said. 'Just a pound.' And shook his head in disbelief.

'You're too softhearted,' I said.

'Pink's Law,' he said, looking me straight in the eye. 'I forgot it, boy, didn't I?'

'It was a greyhound, not a Dalmatian or a leopard,' I reminded him.

'Not the dog, Hugh, the man! Pink's Law can apply to people, too. Never make a diagnosis on one factor alone, remember?'

I nodded several times.

'But I did. I did!' C.J. said, clasping his hands. 'Now remember this, young man.' C.J. tapped his nose gently with his forefinger. 'If they are dirty and scruffy, they could be Micks, on the other hand — they could be millionaires!' Then C.J. Pink threw back his head and roared with laughter.

And for me, that was another section of Pink's Law that proved invaluable, as well.

*   *   *

I spent all my vacations 'seeing practice' at Barrow Hill. Some students moved about a lot and visited a great variety of practices, but I spent my time with C. J. Pink and never regretted one moment of it.

His guidance and advice, together with abundant quotations from 'Pink's Law', put a completely different interpretation upon the final terms at university.

Now, the lectures, clinical demonstrations and surgical procedures were really beginning to mean something. The basic foundation of the first years was at last being built upon in real terms and I was beginning to feel and think like a vet.

But, as the days flew by and the final examinations loomed, there was something nagging at me, that up until then I had successfully banished to the distant corners of my mind — National Service. Even if I qualified, obtained my degree and became a member of the prestigious Royal College of Veterinary Surgeons, I would not be able to go into practice until I had completed two years in the Army. Most graduates took a commission in the Royal Army Veterinary Corps, which dealt with horses and dogs and was certainly no waste of time, but for me it was just an unnecessary delay in achieving my ambition of becoming a country vet.

There are some great crossroads in life that one often fails to recognise at the time, because they do not appear as momentous occasions. Such was one of mine — nothing more dramatic than losing the top of my treasured Parker 51 fountain pen that my parents had given me when I started at university. I searched high and low, then decided to put a 'Lost' card on the notice board outside the student common room.

The board was usually crowded with day-to-day information — everything from time-tables and team lists to club news, entertainments and other oddments of interest. As I scanned the board for a space, I noticed a directive stating that, due to a delay in recruitment, graduates due for National Service would not be called up for at least two months after qualifying. This I regarded as bad news, for as far as I could see, it only delayed the agony.

There appeared to be no spare drawing pins, and as I was desperately hoping to obtain news of my lost pen top, I decided to pinch a pin from some less significant notice. I found one, almost completely obscured by a poster for the Friday Dance, at the bottom corner of the board. No one could see it anyway, so I felt quite justified in taking its pin and fixing my card in a prominent position.

Standing back to admire my bold notice, I casually looked at the card I had just displaced. It was a vacancy for a job. Occasionally these cards appeared on the board, but as I was destined for the Army, I paid little attention to them: the one in my hand, however, captured my interest.

A vacancy exists for a temporary assistant. The practice is mixed agricultural and the position, which would suit a new graduate, is for an approximate period of thirty days.

Apply in the first instance to:

G.R. HACKER MRCVS,
ST MARK'S SQUARE,
LEDINGFORD,
HEREFORDSHIRE

I put the card in my pocket and wrote that night.

I got the job and, when I qualified, started practice in Ledingford. The advert was indeed true to its description, in that the practice was agricultural and very mixed. For thirty days at least, I would be able to satisfy my ambition.

Three

'Thirteen pounds a week and a Ford car, for use when off duty,' was the agreement. But as 'off duty' was only to be one weekend from mid-day Saturday during my stay, it wasn't that much of a perk.

But, I should care! I had made it! I was going to be a country vet, and with youthful enthusiasm and boundless optimism, I stepped off the train at Ledingford station.

Hacker's surgery occupied a most prestigious position in St Mark's Square, in the centre of the town. Ledingford's great antiquity and considerable architectural variety was very evident as I surveyed my first place of employment.

Number One, St Mark's Square was at the centre of a row of stylish Georgian houses facing the Merchants' Hall, the latter being an imposing stone building sporting a pillared façade in Grecian style. To the left stood the Town Hall, also imposing, but of brick and terracotta, with a Renaissance influence. By contrast, the Norman Church of St Mark, with its eleventh century adornments and high pointed spire, completed the surroundings.

Even from across the street, a good hundred yards away, the glistening brass plate outside Number One shone like a beacon, and I homed in on it speedily.

G. R. HACKER MRCVS
VETERINARY SURGEON

The solid oak door was open, revealing a small recess covered with a thick coconut mat, whose rugged texture defied anyone to enter with unclean footwear. To the right and leading off was another door, the upper part panelled with frosted glass.

There were no instructions to ring or knock, but the highly polished brass knob invited to be turned.

This I did, pushing the door at the same time.

It stuck briefly and needed a second shove before it yielded, then it flew open sharply, accompanied by a fierce jangling from above as it triggered off a bell on a curved spring over my head.

Distracted by the deafening alarm, I failed to notice the step and, catching my toe, plunged forward onto my knees. As I fell, the catch of my suitcase caught the big brass knob and snapped open, the contents cascading onto the floor about me. And so it was, on my knees, surrounded by shirts, pants, vests and pyjamas, an open toilet bag and two pairs of shoes, that I made my grand entry into veterinary practice.

The jangling of the bell gradually subsided and, as I recovered from my shock, I became aware of someone standing before me. My gaze slowly ascended, taking in sensible brown lace-up shoes, thick woollen stockings, tweed skirt, long-sleeved brown ribbed jumper, horn-rimmed spectacles, tightly permed hair and a frosty female face.

'Well!' she exclaimed.

Kneeling was never a good position from which to assert oneself, and with my belongings scattered about me I felt like an exploded commercial traveller. In an attempt to regain my composure I scrambled to my feet.

The frosty woman looked me over, as if she was surveying something rather distasteful.

'I'm Hugh Lasgarn, the new veterinary surgeon. I've spent five years at Glasgow where I have studied veterinary medicine and surgery. I have also seen practice with the highly esteemed C. J. Pink, MRCVS, of Newpool. I have been granted my degree of BVMS and I am also, by election, a Member of the Royal College of Veterinary Surgeons!'

Well, that's what I should have said; actually what I did

say was:

'I'm Hugh Lasgarn and I've come to h-help out,' and I even said that rather weakly.

The frosty woman sniffed.

'You should have been here this morning,' she snapped icily. 'Mr Hacker Senior went into hospital last night. Both young Mr Hacker and Mr McBean are on farm visits.' She breathed in deeply, so that the stitches of the ribbed jumper tensed uneasily, and then added curtly, 'And I have an emergency!' With that she turned on her heel and disappeared behind a partition that screened one corner of the room.

For the first time I was able to take stock of my surroundings. The surgery was larger and more purposeful than C. J. Pink's and reminded me rather of a museum. The fittings and furniture were very solid and highly polished. All the cupboards had bright brass catches and hinges, and between them the shelves were lined with a vast number of bottles and jars. Leading from the screened area ran a shining oak counter, on which stood an apothecary's weighing scales and alongside it lay a large ledger. The counter separated the reception area from a small dispensary with white ceramic jars, carrying illuminated Latin inscriptions describing their contents: 'Oleo Cetacei', 'Unguentum Cucumeris', 'Pulv Antimon' and the like. Between these and the counter, and facing the front, was a show case containing instruments. Some, such as whelping forceps, tooth elevators and gags, I recognised, and catheters and dilators were also familiar, but others were models of engineering precision, with chains and wheels and variable screws, defeating even the most flexible imagination as to the reason for their use. Just to my right was a long bench seat and in the corner was fixed a large wash basin. From the wall above sprouted two fearsome taps, looking so powerful that one could easily believe that a jet from their dilated nozzles would quickly expel any debris, bacteria or substance of decay, swiftly down the nearest drain to Hell.

The frosty woman re-appeared from behind the screen. Clasping her hands, she inhaled sharply, the jumper stitches again taking the strain.

'I am Miss Billings,' she announced. 'Mr Hacker Senior's secretary, receptionist and book-keeper. I also dispense medicines, order drugs and assist in the surgery. And you, Mr Lasgarn,' she repeated again, 'should have been here this morning!'

'I said I would come up on Thursday,' I replied. 'I thought I could settle in today and start tomorrow.'

'No time for that,' retorted Miss Billings sharply. 'Both Mr Hacker Junior and Mr McBean are miles away and I've got an emergency. So you'll have to start now. Pick up your belongings and I'll give you instructions.' Then she swept behind the screen for a second time.

Although I was a little peeved at being ordered about like a manservant, the excitement of the emergency had triggered off my adrenalin and I pushed my annoyance to the back of my mind. Here I was at last, qualified and in practice — about to tackle an emergency.

Speedily I rammed my things back into my case, squeezed down the lid and placed it upon the counter.

As if triggered by an invisible switch, as the case touched the wood Miss Billings shot from behind the screen.

'Off!' she shouted. 'Off!'

I looked at her in amazement.

'Off to where?' I asked.

'Your case!' she screeched. 'Off the counter!'

I quickly lifted it up as her head swooped down on the spot. She peered closely, searching for any abrasion on the shining surface. Satisfied that there was no damage, she raised her head and gave me a withering look.

'Nothing! Nothing!' she repeated, her voice scratchy and witch-like, 'is ever placed on Mr Hacker's counter!'

I put my case on the floor and apologised. I'd never really come across a woman of Miss Billings' type before, but even with my limited experience of dragons, I realised that it was best to tread carefully.

But my adrenalin was still high and my enthusiasm undaunted.

'What is the emergency?' I asked manfully. 'I'll handle it.'

At this, Miss Billings relaxed, gave a condescending sniff and consulted the ledger, which was obviously very important, being allowed on the counter.

'It's a cat with a bone in its throat,' she said without raising her eyes. 'Belongs to Mrs Jarvis, Offa's Close. Mr Hacker Senior always attends Mrs Jarvis' cat personally, but as he is indisposed and it is an emergency, she will accept someone else.'

I had always imagined emergencies to be big situations. Cows calving, bulls blown or horses injured — a cat with a bone in its throat didn't seem to have the same kudos.

But to Mrs Jarvis it was no doubt very important — and I would go.

'Where is it?' I asked.

'You can walk,' Miss Billings advised sharply. 'It's only a short way. Go down past the Town Hall and take the first turning left, straight across at the junction and Offa's Close is at the end. Mrs Jarvis lives in number four, they are alms houses and she is old and very deaf.'

'Right!' I said. 'I'll go straight away.'

My hand was on the doorknob, but she called me back.

'Don't you want anything?' she enquired, peering over the tops of her horn-rimmed spectacles.

'Want anything?' I replied, slightly puzzled.

'The others usually take a case, with drugs and instruments.'

I released the knob and stepped back towards the sacred counter.

'I'll see what I can find,' she said, and disappeared through the door into another room.

In a few minutes she returned carrying a very smart leather medical case, which she held towards me, but just before I could take it, she withdrew it slightly.

'You have not been allocated any equipment. Mr Hacker

71

Junior will do that when he returns. I shouldn't really be doing this, but it's an emergency and I suppose it will be all right.' Then she inhaled deeply and the jumper stitches tensed again. 'This case belongs to Mr Hacker Senior. It will contain all you need, but take exceptional care of it and return it to me as soon as you come back.'

As she presented it to me I was tempted to shake her hand, such was the drama of the moment, but I thought better of it. In fact, it *was* rather a special occasion, in that here I was, green as grass, going to my first emergency, armed with the case belonging to an illustrious and highly respected veterinarian. Who could have asked for a more momentous initiation into the profession?

To the sound of the clanging bell, I left the surgery, carefully negotiating the step and closing the door firmly behind me. I didn't glance back at Miss Billings, but put my best foot forward to minister unto Mrs Jarvis' cat.

Offa's Close was a group of alms houses which could only be described as quaint. They were set in a quadrangle whose centre was a mixture of rosebeds and grassy places divided by pavestone walkways. Two willow trees and a tidy beech gave shade to the occasional wooden seats.

The dwellings were single storey and built of stone, with delicate lattice windows and studded oak doors. Eight in all, four pairs, and Number Four was Mrs Jarvis.

I rapped the wrought iron knocker confidently, then stood back, clasping G. R. Hacker's case in front of me. While no movement came from within, I was conscious of being observed from all sides, yet when I turned quickly there was no one, just an occasional quiver of a curtain behind a few of the lattice windows. Just as I was about to knock again I heard a shuffling and gasping, then the flap of the letterbox in the door disappeared inwards and I saw a pair of eyes replace it.

'Mrs Jarvis!' I shouted. But the eyes remained immobile. 'The vet, Mrs Jarvis. I've come to see your cat.'

The flap closed and there followed a great creaking and

drawing of bolts. Then the studded oak door slowly opened and Mrs Jarvis came into view.

She was a typical 'little old lady', grey haired, bespectacled, a dark woollen shawl about her shoulders. She looked up at me and smiled, then turned away and motioned me to follow.

Mrs Jarvis led me into her living room, which again was quaint and just what one might have expected a 'little old lady' to live in. Neat, chintzy, with the minimum of walking space, it was more a collection of memories than a habitation. On a mahogany sideboard along one wall was displayed an array of photographs of family, soldiers, nurses, dogs, cats, young people on bicycles, seaside snapshots and the Royal Family. Lustre jugs, willow pattern plates, a boy holding cherries over his head, an Alsatian dog looking skywards, tiny teapots and a cheese dish completed the display.

A square table occupied the centre, covered with a red woollen cloth with tassels around its border.

But the most eye-catching feature of Mrs Jarvis' homestead was the fireplace. Not just for the pleasant glow of the coals, but complementing the brightness and the warmth of the room was a row of brass candlesticks that surmounted the tall mantelshelf. I had never seen so many in one collection before, ranging from thumbnail size, graduating evenly to a centrepiece at least twelve inches in height, each one balanced by its partner on the opposite side. There must have been fifty in all.

I placed my case, or rather Mr Hacker's case, on the table. Momentarily, I checked myself, for the last time I had put my case on a table I had been swiftly admonished, but this time there was no reproach.

'I blame myself,' said Mrs Jarvis meekly. 'All because I didn't look. You see, it's very rarely I have salmon, but we were all given a piece by the Fishing Club and I left it on the table to cool. Samson jumped up and took it, and the next thing I knew he was choking. He spat and rubbed his mouth and I was so distressed, I didn't know what to do, but then the Vicar called and saw what had happened, so he phoned Mr Hacker.'

'I'm sorry,' I said, 'but Mr Hacker has gone to hospital, so I have come instead.'

'Poor Mr Hacker,' she said. 'Such a gentleman.'

'Well now, Mrs Jarvis.' I began to look for my patient. 'Where's the cat?'

She bent down and raised the edge of the red cloth, which hung quite low around the table.

'There he is,' she cooed. 'There's my Samson. Come out dear, where we can see you.'

In the semi-darkness between the table legs I saw two bright green eyes staring keenly at me. Gradually, as I accustomed to the half light, Samson's body took shape. He was not as large as his name might have suggested, but his coat was sleek and his movements agile and he came forward in response to Mrs Jarvis' call. I could see that his mouth was unnaturally half open and his jaws appeared locked, but despite the inconvenience, he still managed to hiss aggressively.

'No, it's not Mr Hacker,' said Mrs Jarvis, addressing Samson, 'it's the other gentleman, Mr . . .'

'Lasgarn, Hugh,' I prompted.

'It's Mr Lasgarnew,' she repeated. 'Are you foreign?' she asked, turning to me.

'Welsh,' I said.

But the information didn't impress Samson at all as, still hissing through his jammed mouth, he leaped onto an armchair and sat on the cushion in a guarded manner.

'Perhaps I can take a closer look,' I offered and made a move forward, but Samson was ready and stood up immediately as if to make a quick departure.

'Now don't be silly,' reprimanded Mrs Jarvis, approaching her cat and wagging her finger at him. 'Mr Lasgarnew wants to help you. Sorry about this,' she added demurely. 'Normally he's quite good, but when he wants to, he can be a real bugger!'

Before I could even raise my eyebrows, she had grabbed

Samson and quite unceremoniously lifted him onto the table.

I quickly steadied him by grasping his scruff, forcing him downwards, and he lay still, submitting to the pressure.

'Are you all right?' I shouted to Mrs Jarvis.

'Yes,' she replied, her face grim with concentration. 'I can manage this end for you.'

'Thanks,' I said, thinking to myself that there was more to this sweet little old lady than met the eye. 'Now let's have a look at his mouth.' Still holding firmly to his scruff, I extended my grip to clamp my thumb and forefinger either side of Samson's head. As I rotated it gradually, putting pressure on the angle of his jaws, with my other hand I slowly depressed his lower jaw. Samson moaned evilly but did not resist, and as I widened the aperture I saw, jammed across the top of his mouth, a thin spicule of fishbone.

'I can see it,' I said. 'Next thing is to get it out.' I decided that this was no finger operation, as Samson's teeth were needle-sharp and his attitude unco-operative to say the least.

'If you can hang on,' I shouted, 'I'll see if there is an instrument in the case.'

Mrs Jarvis nodded and her scrawny hands tensed with effort as she restrained Samson.

Mr Hacker's case, when open, revealed three drawers. The lower one contained bottles of injections and pills, the middle one, syringes, a thermometer and a black stethoscope, while in the top one were surgical instruments for suturing wounds.

My eye fell upon a long thin artery forceps, somewhat like a pair of scissors, but with ridged jaws instead of blades. Just the thing, and taking the instrument I again grasped Samson's head and squeezed his cheeks. His moaning increased in volume, but he did not resist unduly, and I was able to get a good grip on the bone. But pulling it out was another matter. Despite a firm tug, it wouldn't budge. Three times I tried, but it was solidly wedged.

'I don't think it's going to come,' I commented loudly.

'Oh, dear!' exclaimed Mrs Jarvis, and with that took her hands away from the sleek black body.   .

Samson needed no further invitation to escape. In a flash his whole body tensed and with claws extended, he drew backwards, cagging the red tasselled tablecloth as he went. As soon as he was beyond my grasp he changed direction and charged forward, scrambling over Mr Hacker's medical case which unbalanced and, with the drawers sliding out, discharged all the medical aids onto the floor. The red tasselled tablecloth followed it. But Samson was clear and in full flight as, like greased lightning, he leaped onto the mahogany sideboard. Pictures and pots went flying, the lid of the cheese dish came adrift, the Alsatian, still staring skywards, was swung round violently and the boy lost his cherries.

Mrs Jarvis and I watched helplessly as Samson continued his career of destruction by leaping onto the curtains. Momentarily his claws held him firm, but his weight was too much for the rail and down came the lot; yet before either of us could make a move, he had miraculously extricated himself and climbed back onto the windowsill.

Shooting a hateful glance at me, he spat loudly, then soared through the air to land on the back of the armchair where he sat and cocked his head quizzically, as if to say, 'Want to see any more?' Then, with an evil smirk on his pointed black face, he looked up at the mantelshelf, on which stood the fifty brass candlesticks, arranged in ascending and descending order.

'Oh, no! Samson!' I shouted. 'Not up there!'

I am sure the black devil winked at me first, before executing a perfectly measured leap from the armchair to the edge of the mantelshelf, and with one defiant look at me ran the length of the line, peeling every single one of the brass candlesticks from its perch as neatly as a set of collapsing dominoes.

Down they came, small ones, large ones, largest one and down the line again. One by one, they hit the cast iron fender and the pokers and tongs with an almighty continuous clatter that would have awakened the dead. Even Mrs Jarvis, deaf as she was, put her hands to her ears.

When the pandemonium subsided and everything had stopped moving I looked about for the black villain, only to discover him sitting quietly beneath the table, whence he had first started, cleaning his paws.

I turned to face Mrs Jarvis, not knowing what to expect or what to say, and to my profound amazement discovered her to be smiling.

'Thank you so much,' she said. 'Sorry he was naughty.'

'But, I haven't...' I started. Then I realised that if Samson was licking his paws, the bone must have shifted and, looking at the forceps, I discovered the offending obstruction clamped firmly between its jaws.

The devastation did not seem to perturb Mrs Jarvis in any way, and when I offered to replace the candlesticks she said she would clean them first, and that it had saved her the bother of getting down, as being so short she found it quite difficult. I re-assembled Mr Hacker's case and collected up the contents. To my sheer good fortune it appeared undamaged. All the while Samson maintained his position and warily watched my every movement.

Mrs Jarvis returned from the kitchen.

'I'm sorry to hear about Mr Hacker's indisposition, Mr Lasgarnew,' she said. 'I do hope it's nothing serious.'

'Something to do with his throat, I believe,' I explained. 'He's been intending to have it seen to for some time. That's why I am here, to help out.'

'Do give him this.' She held up a small jar of pickled onions. 'And wish him all the best from Samson and me.'

I thanked her and, taking my case, made for the door.

'I shall tell Mr Hacker how clever you were, when next I see him,' she said, as she closed the door. And I felt rather pleased.

But Mr Hacker never knew, for although he had come through the operation quite well, he suffered a sudden relapse and, following a cardiac arrest, he died that night.

*   *   *

That tragic and completely unexpected event made all the difference to my starting work, for although when I returned to the surgery after the fishbone episode and met Mr Hacker Junior, who sorted out my equipment and introduced me to LCJ 186, my Ford car, I saw little of him for the next fortnight. There was much confusion in the practice following the news; Miss Billings, however, who had been terribly shocked and upset, completely altered her attitude to me and became most helpful and co-operative.

But it was McBean who was a pillar of strength and a tremendous aid to me in those early days, taking the lion's share of the work, while I saw the occasional dog and cat in the surgery or handled straightforward jobs, such as lame cows, coughing calves, pigs off their food and horses with mild colic.

McBean was a Belfast Irishman who had qualified from university some six years before me and had spent five of them in Ledingford. Short and stocky, he spoke with a deep Irish brogue, prefacing nearly every statement with 'Well, now!' His manner of dress was more casual than untidy, showing a preference for ex-army purchases at bargain prices. To this effect he sported khaki shirts and trousers and heavy boots, adding colour with a Fair Isle pullover and green tweed jacket. The other constant feature was a flat cap which he wore at a rakish angle.

One advantage from Mr Hacker's unfortunate demise was that I was readily accepted by the clients, who were so upset at what had happened that, for the first few days, they never really questioned my inexperience and mostly seemed reasonably satisfied with my diagnosis and treatment. I bowled around in my little Ford car, feeling on top of the world and so very, very happy.

But my confidence was severely tested when, early in my first week, McBean asked me to go to Donhill Court.

'Well, now!' he began. 'Paxton of Donhill is a very influential and wealthy man and a wicked devil to work for! Mr Hacker Senior was the only man who could really handle him, but he'll not be getting him today, however much he rants,' he added somewhat irreverently. 'I will say this though, the man's got a fine pedigree herd, with some really good stock, but he thinks that all we do is sit on our bums and wait for him to ring. Whenever he wants a vet, he wants him yesterday — everything is a dire emergency to Paxton and every cow that's sick is always his best and most valuable beast.' McBean gave a grunt of disgust, then continued. 'Now I've got one hound of a round south of the river, so it's your good fortune to have to take the call, Hugh.' He stroked his straggling moustache thoughtfully. 'But, well, now! It'll be good experience for you,' he finished.

'What is it?' I asked.

'Should be no problem. It's a cow, his best cow no less, with a swelling on her jaw. Now it could be an "actino" — you're familiar with that?'

I nodded, for I had already seen the slow-growing jaw bone infection of cattle, when I was with C. J. Pink.

'Intravenous iodine,' I suggested.

He nodded. 'Make sure it's in the vein. Now, what else could it be?'

'Tooth problem?'

'Possible,' he agreed.

'Abscess?'

'Yes,' said McBean emphatically. 'Yes. Yes. In fact that's what Big Head Paxton thinks it is. Of course, he always knows better than anyone else. But remember this, Hugh; you've trained for five years on animal symptoms and diseases and so, no matter what buck he gives you, you make your own diagnosis and stick to it. Don't get upset by his attitude — you know more than he does. Good luck to you, now!'

I pondered McBean's remarks as I drove out of the city. The directions to Donhill Court were quite clear: five miles north of Easthope, through the village for another two miles, passing an old quarry on the left, and the farmstead was just beyond it, standing grandly upon a ridge about a quarter of a mile from the road.

From the moment the car crossed the well-maintained cattle grid that guarded the wide entrance to a pot-hole-free, asphalt driveway leading through the meadows, I could tell that Donhill Court was exceedingly well run. Hedges were trim, with no gaps, and the fences firm and tidy. A group of lively but inquisitive Hereford heifers kicked their heels and followed the car at a gallop on the other side of the rails, to the edge of their pasture.

Nearer the buildings the road began to rise and then forked, the left-hand route running to the residence, which was set apart from the buildings and very impressive. It was a large house, brick built and three storeys tall, with panelled windows peeping through a well established Virgina creeper that adorned the front and near side. French windows with lined red velvet curtains led out to a terrace overlooking a grass tennis court, while a sloping porchway at the front appeared to be full of exotic plants and gave access to a well-tended rose garden.

The right fork, which I took, led to a large open yard. I drove in, taking a wide sweep — the little Ford's turning circle not being all that tight — to finish up facing the direction I had come. At least, I thought to myself, I could make a reasonably quick get-away if necessary.

As I swung round, my eye caught Mr Paxton talking to a thin-faced fellow in a lumpy cap and brown stock coat. Talking seemed rather a weak description of the action; from the domineering attitude of the larger man, it appeared to be more of an ultimatum. In fact, it was for that reason that I assumed the aggressor was Mr Paxton.

He gave the impression that he was either leaving for, or had just returned from a funeral or some other formal occasion, for he was clad in a bowler hat, black city coat with a rose in the buttonhole and shining black shoes. In his hand he grasped a silver-topped cane, which he persistently tapped on the ground. I was later to learn that he attired himself thus for most of the year, the only concession to warmer weather being to remove the overcoat, revealing a black suit beneath.

As I drew to a halt, he concluded his chastisement of the unfortunate fellow in the brown stock coat and turned his attention to me.

Taking a deep breath, I got out of the car and slammed the door confidently. The little Ford shuddered at the shock and the bottles in the boot jangled together rather cheaply. Clearing my throat, I walked over to him.

'Mr Paxton?'

He stopped tapping his cane and screwed up his eyes. For the first time I noticed his great bushy eyebrows that seemed to disappear in a rather devilish fashion under his bowler hat.

'Who are you?' he roared.

'Hugh Lasgarn. Mr Hacker ... the late Mr Hacker's assistant,' I replied.

'My God!' said Paxton, still scrutinising me keenly. 'You come by yourself?'

It was pretty obvious that I had. It was a baited question and I felt my neck go a little cold.

'How long have you been qualified, then?' Paxton placed both hands on his cane and rocked back slightly on his heels. This was another testing question, but I came back quickly.

'Long enough,' I replied.

He didn't follow up his enquiry, but changed the line of his interrogation.

'Where's young Hacker?'

'Busy with arrangements.'

'McBean?'

'Has a lot of work south of the river.'

Paxton started to breathe heavily; his face darkened and

his jugulars bulged like drainpipes.

'This won't do!' he shouted, banging the cane on the ground. 'This won't do! I pay that firm a fortune every year and I expect service. Experienced service!' He glared directly at me, his eyes showing red. 'There are other vets, you know,' he stormed, waving the cane about, so that the brown-coated stockman, who had been standing nervously by, took a step backward. 'Other vets who'd only be too ready to do my work!' He really did look evil as he rested his cane on the ground again, his thumb twitching involuntarily on the silver knob.

'It's very unfortunate circumstances,' I said, trying to make my voice firm. But in the face of the unwarranted tirade, my throat had become dry. 'Mr Hacker will be a great loss to the farmers.'

'Farmers!' he bawled arrogantly, as if he were a class above. 'Farmers! That doesn't help me!'

He turned and was about to stalk away. What a pig of a man this is, I thought. My temper rose and my voice, though raised, came firm and clear.

'Nobody could help you!' I shouted after him angrily.

It stopped him in his tracks. He didn't face me immediately, he just stood, staring at the ground. Then, suddenly, he turned and raised his cane. This was great, I thought, two days in practice and about to be slung off a farm. But I was wrong, for Paxton pointed the cane at his man and said:

'Mason, show him the cow.'

The stockman gave him a subservient bow. Then, with a nod of his thin head, he beckoned me to follow.

The farm really was a showpiece, with not a door unpainted, brick out of place or the slightest smell of anything remotely relating to livestock. Two long avenues led from the yard, each one lined by looseboxes, very much in the manner of a racing stable.

But the occupants were all bulls, some of whom pushed their great heads out over the doors and snorted belligerently as we passed, obviously having the same attitude to life as their owner.

Mason opened a door at the end of the row and went inside. I followed him into a spotlessly clean and airy box, to find, standing knee-deep in golden straw, a large placid Hereford cow with a lump on the right side of her face.

'This is 'er,' Mason said, the first time he had uttered a word. 'Oyster Maiden the Third. One of the best.'

'Her first two calves were champions and she's a champion herself!' It was Paxton, who had followed us and was leaning over the door. 'I want to show her this season and I don't want her messed about, d'you understand? Lance it deep and clean, and I don't want any scar to show!'

Mason slipped a white cotton rope halter over Oyster's head and pulled her around for me to see. The swelling was quite obvious, about the size of a small apple, situated midway between the chin and the angle of the lower right jaw.

'I want no fiddling and poulticing with this,' continued Paxton. 'I want it cleared up!'

'How long has she had it?' I enquired.

'How long, Mason?' Paxton roared.

'About . . . about two or three days, boss,' he stuttered nervously. 'Come up quite quick, it did.'

'Can she eat?' I asked.

'Can she eat, Mason?' came the loud echo.

'Yes. Yes, I think so, boss.' Mason's hand shook at the end of the halter.

'Think so! Think so!' bellowed Paxton. 'Yes or no, man?'

'Yes! Yes!' Mason was now visibly quaking.

'Hold her steady,' I said. 'I want to feel it.'

Gently I ran my fingers over and around the protuberance. Oyster Maiden the Third made no movement when I touched it and, even when I pressed it hard, showed no sign of distress. The sides felt fairly firm, but the top was softer, as if it was coming to a head; yet there was no heat in it.

'Seems a bit low for a tooth problem and as it's come up

83

so quickly, it's most unlikely to be "Lumpy Jaw",' I commented, 'Lumpy Jaw' being the colloquial term for an 'actino'.

'Don't start "umming"' and "aaring",' said Paxton impatiently. 'It's an abscess and wants lancing!'

I studied the lump more closely. I really wasn't very keen to lance it as I would need to cut very deep and the chances of healing without a blemish would be slim. If it was given time and allowed to burst naturally it would be safer and more likely to heal better, but with Paxton breathing down my neck I had to try and be positive. Of course, the fact that I was only there for thirty days might let me off the hook, for I would be far away by the show season anyway — but that philosophy didn't suit. I could feel the old tyrant's influence pressurising me, so I decided to play for time.

'I'd like to feel inside the mouth,' I said finally. 'Just to check on the lining of the cheek.'

'You can see it's an abscess, man!' Paxton snapped. 'What more do you want?'

'I'll get a gag,' I said, ignoring his comment, and pushed the half door, forcing him to move. I went back to the car to get the instrument and also to collect my thoughts. 'No matter what buck he gives you, you know more than he does,' McBean had said. At that precise moment, I wasn't too sure. But even so, I was determined not to be rushed.

Drinkwater's gag is an extremely useful piece of veterinary equipment and can save the fingers from being badly damaged when examining a bovine mouth. Although a cow has no upper front teeth, the upper back teeth are present and, in conjunction with the lower ones, form a very efficient grinding machine.

The gag is simple in design, being fashioned from aluminium and about the size of a hand. Oval at one end, to fit at the back of the mouth between the jaws, it has a grooved top and bottom to accommodate the upper and lower molar teeth on the side opposite to the one being examined, rather like a wedge.

With Mason holding Oyster's head firmly with the halter, I slipped the gag between her left jaws. She took it well and, after a bit of a shuffle, stood quietly with her mouth jammed open. Rolling up my sleeves, I grasped the rough slippery tongue and examined the gums of that side, which felt perfectly normal; but when I probed a little further I made a most extraordinary discovery. There was a swelling all right, but it was quite independent of the cheek, teeth or gums. In fact, my fingers were able to run right round it. When I squeezed it, it depressed and when I pulled it — it came away in my hand.

Gradually I withdrew my arm to bring the object into sight. Mason blinked incredulously at what he saw.

'Abscess?' grunted Paxton, from behind. For, with my back to him, he had been unable to see what was going on.

'No, Mr Paxton. It isn't!' I said, still with my back to him.

'What d'yer mean, "It isn't"!' he retorted grumpily.

I turned to face him and held up my find.

'It's a tennis ball!'

Paxton's eyes nearly popped.

'The hair's all gone, but it's a ball all right — jammed between the cheek and the jaw. Good job I didn't lance it, Mr Paxton, isn't it!' Even with my limited experience of practice, I knew I was the winner.

'Where the hell . . . ?' Paxton fumed.

'That bunch have been grazing the paddock next to the tennis lawn for the past week,' said Mason hesitantly.

'Them dam' girls,' raged Paxton. 'I'll stop their games, I will! Mason, you scour that paddock and don't you leave any dam' tennis balls or anything else there. Hear me! That could have choked my best cow! Those nieces of mine will have to be more careful!'

'Lucky escape,' I added, when he went off the boil. 'Could have caused complications, though, if it hadn't been removed.'

'Will she want any more treatment?' asked Paxton.

'I'll leave some drenches for her. There's a bit of bruising where it was stuck and we don't want to take any risks.' I gradually eased the Drinkwater from Oyster's mouth.

'Whatever you say,' said Paxton. 'Give Mason full instructions.'

'I'd like to wash my hands,' I said.

'Mason, get some water. And when you've done . . .' he looked questioningly at me.

'Lasgarn,' I prompted. 'Hugh Lasgarn.'

'Lasgarn,' he repeated. 'You're not foreign?'

'Welsh,' I informed him.

'Same thing,' he grunted. 'I want Lasgarn to look at Warrior — get him out on the yard.' As he stumped off, I collected my things and took them back to the car. Mason arrived shortly with a bucket of hot water, soap and a sparkling white towel, and I washed up.

I was wondering who or what Warrior was, when Mason re-appeared. He was not a small man, but the hulk that he was leading slowly across the yard completely dwarfed him. At the end of a bull rope and staff, clipped into a big brass nose ring, was the largest bull I had ever seen in my life.

One ton of powerful muscle and surging blood, his deep mahogany coat contrasting sharply with the snow white of his magnificent head and crest, while his tail, thick as a tree trunk, flicked relentlessly behind. He approached and lowered his massive head to display a pair of mighty horns. Fearsome weapons if ever they were needed, but there was little doubt, as Warrior rippled his muscular crest and gave an impatient snort from his wide nostrils, that few, if any, would ever dare to challenge this majestic creature.

'This is some bull,' I said, as he turned sideways, casting a shadow over both me and my Ford car. 'He is superb.'

'Walk him around, Mason.' Paxton waved his cane. 'This is my stock bull,' he informed me. 'Finest blood in the breed; his pedigree goes way back to the Grove family. It was a Grove bull that went to America and from him they bred half the cattle in Texas. Fine bull,' he said proudly, as Warrior paraded before us. 'Good worker, hundred per cent fertile and worth a lot of money. There's many as would like to get their hands on Warrior.' He tapped his cane on the ground with a staccato effect. 'Now, Lasgarn, have a good look at him. Tell me what you think.' Paxton started to hum quietly and turned away, as if to detach himself from my examination. I watched Warrior carefully as he moved ponderously about the yard. Taking my time, I followed him up and down several times. I stood ahead of him and watched the movement of his forelimbs; then, I stood behind to check his action at the back.

As if I had been allotted a certain fixed period to come up with the answer, Paxton suddenly cracked the ground with his cane and, swinging round, called, 'Right! What have you to say?'

'Just a minute,' I said, not even looking at the old man. 'Hold him up, Mason, let me have a close look at his feet.'

Mason drew to a halt.

Warrior's feet were clean and well trimmed, but it wasn't difficult to spot the thick folds of tender tissue wedged between his back toes. Even as I watched, the great bull raised one of his feet uneasily and shifted his weight.

'Well?' said Paxton irritably. 'Well?'

'Corns!' I exclaimed. 'He's tender behind.'

'I know that!' The cane banged the ground again. 'What can you do about them?'

'What's been tried?' I asked.

'What have we tried?' Paxton threw back his head and snorted, just like one of his bulls. 'Everything under the sun! Lotions, potions, washes, and ointments. Supplements in the feed, vitamins and even some raspberry leaf tea, which he drank by the gallon!'

Warrior started to paw the ground ominously, as if he was getting rather fed up with the conversation.

'He's worth a lot of money, and if his back end goes — well, he's half the herd, is Warrior. Well, Lasgarn, what do you suggest?'

'It's his tremendous weight,' I said. 'When you think of

the surface area the soles of his feet have to carry, it's not surprising the skin bulges between his toes. When he walks it gets pinched and forms a corn, and the more it grows — the more it hurts.'

'I know all that!' stormed Paxton. 'I've been in cattle since your arse was the size of a shirt button. What I want to know is, as a brand new vet, have you got any brilliant ideas!'

'Cut them out!' I answered.

For a second time that morning Paxton's eyes nearly popped out.

'Cut them out!' he nearly screamed, in such a tone that even Warrior stopped pawing and looked round to see what was going on. 'Cut them out! Are you mad? You're not taking a knife to that bull, I can tell you!' And mumbling fiercely to himself, he took off across the yard in anger.

'You serious?' asked Mason, when the old man had disappeared out of sight.

'I've never seen it done,' I admitted, 'but that's what they recommended at the university.'

'Oh! university!' said Mason, nodding his head, as if that explained everything, and, giving Warrior a gentle tug on the halter, he led the great bull away.

When work had finished that evening, McBean offered to buy me a drink. Over a pint in the Hopman Arms, I told him what had happened at Donhill Court. He listened intently, stroking his moustache and punctuating my story with an occasional 'Well, now!' When I told him how Paxton's eyes popped when I held up the tennis ball, he roared with laughter, slapped his thighs and said:

'Hugh, lad, dear old Hacker would have loved that. What a pity he missed it. Good for you, Hugh!'

'Then he asked me to look at Warrior,' I continued.

'Did he now!' said McBean, his face becoming serious. 'My word, Hugh, you were honoured. Apart from Mr Hacker Senior, no one from this practice has ever been asked to do that.'

'Well, he showed him to me,' I said.

'What was the trouble?' McBean sat up straight on his stool and showed more than passing interest.

'Corns,' I answered.

'Oh, yes,' he said. 'Persistent problem. Mr Hacker tried most things; I suppose the old fart asked you for a cure.'

'Yes, he did,' I replied.

'What did you say?' McBean asked.

'Cut them out!'

'Cut them out?' McBean exploded into the pint pot he was just bringing to his lips. 'You didn't say, "Cut them out", did you?'

I nodded.

'Mother Mary, Hugh! How are you going to do that?'

'With an anaesthetic, of course.'

'Anaesthetic, with a bull of that size?' McBean shook his head. 'Too much of a risk, young man. Too much of a risk. Lord save us, if that Warrior should snuff it while you're cutting away his corns . . .' The Irishman made a spluttering sound and threw his hands up to indicate a bomb exploding. 'Goodbye, Hugh!' His last action reminded me of Talfyn Thomas and the Germans and, thinking it over, I could see that Paxton's reaction under those circumstances would be equally as hostile.

'What did Paxton say?' McBean was now perched precariously, right on the very edge of his stool.

'He said I was mad. And that nobody was going to take a knife to his bull. Then he tore off in a rage.'

'Thank God for that!' McBean rubbed his forehead earnestly. 'That could just have been a bit of a problem.'

'I'm sorry,' I said. 'It was a bit rash to jump in like that.'

'Never mind,' said McBean, 'it's early days yet. But remember, Hugh, what you say, you must be able to back up. Always weigh up the risks versus the results, because in this game they take miracles for granted — they only remember you by your mistakes!'

'I'm a bit green yet,' I said disconsolately.

'Green — not a bit of it,' said McBean, gathering up the glasses. 'Why, when I started, I was so green I thought an "abbattoir" was a French tart's bedroom!' and laughing heartily at his own expense, he bought another round.

*　　　　　*　　　　　*

I took digs with a spinster lady in Church Road, Putsley, about two miles from the surgery, in a substantially built three-bedroomed semi. It had been recommended by McBean and, when I called, I decided it would be most acceptable on two counts. Firstly, the landlady was Welsh, originating from Pembrokeshire, and secondly, because of the sign hanging in her hall. It was in gold lettering on an oblong piece of black wood, hanging next to the hallstand, and it read:

'The more I see of people, the more I like my dog.'

The odd thing was that it was far from apt, for Doris Bradley — or Brad as she was known — loved people and had a heart of gold. Neither did she have a dog, but instead owned two fat and contented cats.

I paid three pounds and ten shillings weekly for bed, breakfast and evening meal, with a bedroom of my own and sharing the lounge and dining room with the other lodger, a Cockney lad of about my own age.

The first night I met him, I thought how alike to Elvis Presley, except that his hair was blond, not black. But the style was the same, curly and profuse at the front, severely slashed back at the sides and heavily greased. He was tall and well built, his shoulders adequately filling his powder-blue drape jacket. Drainpipe trousers, winkle picker shoes, heavily buckled belt and from his neck, filling the gap in his open embroidered shirt, hung a medallion on a gold chain. He pushed out a ringed and braceleted hand.

'Charlie Love's the name,' he announced. 'Love by name and love by nature.'

'Hugh Lasgarn,' I replied, grasping his palm firmly. He had a good handshake, despite his pretty looks.

'Odd moniker that. Where you from?'

'I'm from Wales.'

'Ah! I was in Wales once. Used to go out with a girl from Merthyr Tydfil. Teddy bear stuffer, she was, in a toy factory.' Charlie winked wickedly. 'Oow!! She was a little raver. Lucky ole' teddy bears, eh!' He rubbed his hands warmly together. 'Lumpy old country though, is Wales.'

He then produced a comb from his back trouser pocket and, turning to the mirror over the fire-place, proceeded to sweep it deftly through his greasy locks, following its passage rhythmically with the other hand.

'D'you know why it's so lumpy, Hubert?' he asked, still preening his locks in the mirror.

'Hugh,' I reminded him, but before I could add anything else, he turned about, slid the comb back into his pocket, folded his arms and said: 'Well, my son, I'll tell you.' He took a deep breath. 'Now, no disrespect to you, Hubert,' he began, 'but the Welsh have always been a thieving lot of bas...' he broke off and shook his head sagely. 'Many years ago, they used to come over the wall, raping and pillaging and generally getting up to a bit of nonsense; and amongst doing all sorts of naughty things, they stole a lot of land. Now, when they got it all back home, they found they had too much. So, what did they do?' He eyed me quizzically. 'They piled it all up in heaps, didn't they? That's why you've got so many bleedin' hills down there, Hubert. Surely you know that?'

Charlie tried hard to keep a straight face, but he couldn't for long and broke into raucous laughter, subsiding with a flop into an adjacent armchair. Then he pulled out a packet of Player's from the breast pocket of his embroidered shirt.

'Smoke, Hubert?' He offered one up.

I shook my head. 'No thanks.' Charlie then took what appeared to be a gold lighter and, with a great flourish, lit up, closed his eyes, inhaled, then, taking the cigarette from his lips, blew a great stream of grey-blue smoke into the air.

'You're a vet, Brad tells me,' he continued. 'Bit in the

91

same way myself.'

'What's that?' I asked with interest, wondering what occupation this city character and I could possibly have in common.

'Butchery!' he replied, grinning. 'Presentation of the finished article, you might say.'

I would never have guessed.

'The guv'nor I work for is very, very sharp.' Charlie tapped his nose with his right-hand index finger in the manner of C. J. Pink, although there the resemblance ended. 'Setting up butcher's shops all over, he is. I come down to give it the treatment. Get it going — "Love the Shove", you might say, an' then of course you might not.' He dragged deeply on his cigarette. 'It's the old chat that gets them going; they love the patter: "'Owe abart a bit o' skirt then, darlin'!"' he shouted out. '"Try some of our sausages — keep your old man on his toes!"' There was not doubt about it, I could see he had the touch.

'Then, when it's ticking over nice, I move on to the next one.' His face took on the satisfied look of a man who knew he was a success and, from the way he chirped on, I could see why the housewives loved it.

But as well as the chat and the Teddy Boy style, Charlie was a grafter, out at six every morning and often back after me at night.

It was because of Charlie that we ate well at Brad's, for he often brought home steak, chops or sausages from his work and would never let Brad or me pay anything towards it. The more I got to know him, the more I liked his extrovert ways; his jokes and constant chatter, and his individual approach to life, were in such contrast to what I was beginning to find in Herefordshire.

The practice was very extensive and took in a wide variety of agricultural husbandry: from the Black Mountains in the west, with ancient stone farmsteads, mountain sheep and wild ponies — where everyone was either a Morgan, a Powell or a Watkins — to the lush watermeadows along the river and the hop farms to the east.

Hop farms were new to me and reminiscent of the stories I had read about the cotton plantations of the Deep South of America. They were expansive properties with grand, imposing residences, solid, red-bricked barns, cattle yards and pinnacle-roofed kilns. The hop yards stretched for miles over gently undulating countryside, dormant and naked in winter, awaiting spring when, flushing green, the bines would swarm the poles in flourishing growth.

Hop farming families, too, were old-established, ruling their fertile empires not unlike eastern potentates. The owners were often large, red faced and jolly, their wives well-dressed and haughty, their sons wild and the daughters pretty.

The workers, too, were also long-established. Bent, animal-wise cowmen, knowledgeable shepherds; strong young farm-hands, father followed by son, as in the grand houses were the cooks and the maids, daughter following mother.

'Master' and 'Mistress' were still accepted titles, but without any subservience by their staff; it just came naturally, through long-standing respect and loyalty.

It was, indeed, like going back several decades, and during my childhood in Abergranog and my student days at Glasgow University, I had never realised that such relationships and life-styles still existed.

The livestock reflected the rich and fertile living, with magnificent pedigree Herefords, fat Clun and Kerry sheep and fine thoroughbred horses grazing the pastures. Orchards abounded with low-slung trees, that in their time gave fruit to eat and fruit to crush for cider — another of the county's famous products that I was soon to taste and learn to respect.

Red earth, red cattle, red apples — that was the pattern, and in the early days, as I wended my way through the highways and byways, over hump-backed bridges and mountain tracks, I realised that it was everything a country vet could wish for.

Doris Bradley was in her early fifties, dark-haired, full-figured and pleasant. She was usually attired in print dresses that she made herself, tightly gathered at the waist, short ankle socks and sandals. Her mode of transport was a green Raleigh bicycle with a three-speed hub. She only ever used the bottom gear which was very low, so that her legs would make at least ten turns to every yard and she would appear to be peddling fast but going nowhere.

But Brad cared for us with sincere dedication, like a second mother. Her life had already been one of service devoted to her parents, who had suffered ill health for a considerable time and had both died a few years previously. With little savings and no income, taking in lodgers had become a necessity.

She had never married, but had been engaged in the early forties to a young naval officer whose photo, showing him smartly attired in uniform with cap under arm, stood in a silver frame in the centre of the sideboard. But his ship had been torpedoed in the Atlantic and all hands lost.

To this day, I have never really appreciated what a good soul she was, for apart from looking after Charlie and myself, she cleaned and carried for several old folk nearby and was always visiting the sick, or sewing and washing for someone in need. To me she gave a '24-hour' service, and well do I remember my first night on duty.

It was the Saturday at the end of my first full week and Mr Hacker Senior's son, Bob, who was now head of the practice, asked me if I would be on call. I stayed up until eleven, then decided to go to bed and was soon in a deep sleep.

I was awakened by a jogging movement at my left shoulder; at first I shook it off and tried to settle down, but it persisted and I turned over and opened my eyes.

It was Brad in her night attire:

'The 'phone, Mr Lasgarn. It's Mr Hacker!'

I took a little time to get orientated and was still not quite with it when I reached the hallway and picked up the receiver.

'That you, Hugh?' It was Bob Hacker's voice.

'Yes, it's me,' I replied.

'You all right?' he asked.

'Yes, fine. I just woke up a bit quickly, that's all.'

'Sorry,' he said. 'One of the pleasures of being a vet.' I didn't quite appreciate his sense of humour at the time and he continued: 'Amos Breeze at Gwyllicwmbach has got a cow down. Sounds like a milk fever, she calved yesterday. Can you handle it?'

'Gwylli . . . where?' I asked.

'Gwyllicwmbach, down towards your country. Take the Abergavenny road to Pendulas, turn sharp left by the Council offices, up the hill for about a mile and you'll see a barn by the roadside; then you pass a telephone box on the right. Go on down the slope and turn left at the bottom, and two hundred yards on turn sharp right, then up the lane to Sunnybank Farm.'

I hastily scribbled the directions on the pad.

'Nice old boy,' Bob Hacker added. 'Lives on his own. Manage it all right?'

'Yes, sure,' I replied, feeling far more awake.

'Good luck!' said Bob and clicked off.

'I've made some coffee and cut some sandwiches for you. Now I'll go and open the front gates,' said Brad from the kitchen doorway. 'What a shame you have to go out at this time of night.'

'One of the pleasures of being a vet,' I replied, and thanked her for waking me. 'But I can do the gates.'

'You go and change,' she said and, as I went back upstairs, I thought how kind-hearted she was and what a wonderful wife she would have made that poor lost sailor.

The little Ford obliged by starting first pull. At just on midnight its co-operation was very welcome, for it could be a bit obstinate at times, having already endured over 40,000 veterinary miles in the hands of McBean, who had now graduated to a more modern Ford Prefect.

'Veterinary miles are different from ordinary miles,' McBean told me once, 'and to be driven by a vet is a unique experience for any car. It's no myth that vets aren't like ordinary drivers. You see, it all stems from early training when everything was related to the horse.' He then expounded his theory.

'There was a time when our profession consisted solely of horse doctors, rather than vets. Although, there's a very great difference between doctoring and vetting, as any self-respecting tom cat will tell you,' he added with a chuckle. 'But although our outlook with respect to livestock has changed, our relationship with the horse is still very strong and that's why vets' driving style is so special. They don't just sit there and steer, they drive as they would ride a horse, urging the cars on, coaxing them up hills, easing them around bends and skidding them to a halt. You watch a vet drive: he sits on the edge of his seat, crouching lightly over the wheel to keep his centre of gravity forward, like riding a racehorse. If he overtakes, you'll notice he gives only a fleeting glance to the opposition as he forces his mount forward. Of course,' he concluded, 'my theory also explains why you often see vets' cars perched on hedges or upside-down in ditches, because they sometimes get carried away; they think they are at a point-to-point!'

I smiled to myself as I drove along the Abergavenny road when I thought of McBean's theory; there was no doubt about it, vets did drive differently, and my mind went back to C. J. Pink, who manoeuvred his car in a series of straight lines, driving sedately at thirty miles an hour on main roads and about eighty around farm lanes.

Little LCJ 186 was my first car and, even in the short time I had driven it, I had come to realise that it had a personality all its own. It was not very stylish, being more of a 'sit up and beg' type of design; black with two doors and quite high off the ground, which was an advantage around the rutted tracks. Being a utility model, there were no refinements, no heater or washers. I remember asking McBean what the potatoes were for in the parcel shelf, thinking I was being humorous; I was quite taken aback when he explained that, if the windscreen should freeze, a potato cut in half and rubbed on the outside would clear it. He then showed me how it was possible to do this while in motion, by curling the right arm through the passenger window and on to the front to act like an extra windscreen wiper.

After a few days I had to agree with him that, not only did vets drive their cars like jockeys, but the cars responded like horses — at least my little Ford did! It actually leaped over hump-backed bridges, of which there were quite a few, completely leaving the ground to land with a bump on all fours, or wheels — while I came down next, and the kit landed last, with a great crash.

That night, however, we buzzed along merrily with no leaps or bucks, for the road was smooth, even though the night was very dark. So black was it, that there was absolutely nothing to be seen beyond the thin gleam of the two wing-mounted headlamps. The countryside was indeed fast asleep.

In Pendulas, even the garage and shop were in darkness, and as I turned up the hill by the Council offices, there was not a light anywhere in the village. When I had gone about a mile, I began to look for the barn, but it was difficult to discern anything other than the roadside verge and the butts of the hedges. I wondered if I had missed it and kept my eyes skinned for the telephone box, which was the next clue and should be more obvious; but nothing came into view.

I slowed down and took every bend more cautiously but without any success, and after about two miles I stopped and had to admit I was lost.

Pitch black, depths of the countryside, dead of night — not a place for the faint-hearted. What, I wondered, was my next move? I had a choice: either I could go back to Pendulas, although I was sure I had taken the right road from there, or I could go on in hope.

I decided to carry on.

My spirits rose when, around the next bend, I saw a cottage showing a light in an upstairs window. I pulled up outside, got out and popped in through the garden gate to the front door. There was no bell or knocker, so I hammered on the wood with my fist. As soon as I did so, the light went out. All became silent, so I hammered again, but with no response. Then I shouted:

'I'm the vet! I want to get to Sunnybank Farm. Can you tell me the way, please?'

But it was to no avail. Silent as the grave. Gone to ground, as they say in hunting circles. As I fastened the gate and returned to my car, I decided that the occupants were not so unco-operative after all, because who, in their right mind, in the middle of the countryside at night, would answer the door to a stranger, even if he said he was a vet? Perhaps if I'd said I was a vicar or a policeman, or even Elvis Presley, they might have listened. But they didn't, and that was that.

To my relief and surprise, around the next bend was another cottage and again it had a light in an upstairs window. There was no question about it, I had to give it another try.

Approaching the door, I wondered if I should alter my tactics, but there was a bold brass knocker in the centre; I dispensed with intrigue and banged the door vigorously.

To my delight, the cottage did not go into darkness; instead, there was a great banging and scraping, as if some heavy furniture was being dragged across the floor. This was followed by what sounded like at least six doors slamming one after the other, then there came a crash, like glass shattering, and heavy footsteps coming down a hollow staircase. Keys were turned and bolts drawn, there was much grunting and heavy breathing and the door, with a reluctant shudder, partly opened. A small paraffin lamp came through the gap first; it spluttered and spat, so that the light it gave came in flashes rather than a steady glow.

The face that followed was difficult to age. It was male, mustachioed and rather pale. Below it, in half silhouette, the body appeared to be clad in white combinations; as for feet, I couldn't tell, for the light didn't reach that far.

'I'm the vet from Ledingford,' I explained. 'I'm looking for Mr Breeze at Sunnybank Farm. I was given directions, but I must have gone wrong somewhere. Can you help me?'

The man didn't reply, but just kept staring at me through the intermittent rays of the lamp.

'I came up from Pendulas,' I continued, 'and I was told to look for a barn by the roadside, then a telephone box, and to turn left at the bottom of the slope — but I didn't see any of them.'

Still the man didn't utter a word.

'Can you help me?' I pleaded.

Suddenly his expression altered and he smiled.

'Help me! Help me!' he said, nodding his head up and down.

'You can?' I asked, hopefully.

'No, help me! I Polish. No English. Goodnight!' And with that, he shut the door.

Despondently, I walked back to the car. Just my luck: the whole of Herefordshire in the middle of the night, only one bloke awake — and he had to be a foreigner!

I slammed the door and pulled the starter. The little Ford zipped into life, for which I was very grateful. It really would have been the last straw if the engine had failed. I drove on for about ten minutes until I came to a T-junction pointing in the direction in which I had come. It said, 'Pendulas — 5 miles'. I had obviously come too far.

Turning about, I set off back, but this time carefully noting the mileage. Bob Hacker had said that I should turn left at the bottom of the slope about a mile from the village;

now that I was going in the opposite direction, I would have to turn right at the beginning of a hill about three miles away. After just under three miles, I did meet a hill and, to my great relief, there was a turning sharp right.

It led into a lane, and at the head of it was an opening, beside which was a broken gate, leaning against a low wall. The lights of the little Ford panned across it, illuminating, in faded white lettering,

'SUNNYBANK FARM.'

Foot down, I urged the car onwards and up the rough and rutted lane into a yard, which was in no better condition. But it didn't matter; it was Sunnybank Farm and that was the main thing.

The farm cottage was at the far end of the buildings, and as I approached, I could see Amos Breeze standing with a tilly lamp in the porchway. Squelching to a halt in the mud, I got out and, as I did, he came forward to meet me.

'Hullo, Mr Hacker. Good of you to come. Sorry to hear about your father.'

As Amos came nearer, he raised the lamp and screwed up his eyes. 'T'ain't Mr Hacker. Now who be you, then?' he asked suspiciously.

'Hugh Lasgarn. Mr Hacker's new assistant,' I explained.

'Mr Lasgarn. Mr Hacker's assistant,' Amos repeated vaguely.

'Had a bit of a job finding you,' I said.

'Oh,' said Amos, somewhat mystified, 'now why should that be? Hacker's have been coming 'ere for years.'

'I was told to look out for a barn by the roadside,' I replied.

'Burnt down last month.'

'Then there was the telephone box.'

'Moved it on Wednesday to the Cross.'

'And I stopped at a cottage to ask and a Pole answered the door.'

'That would be Jack Gibbon's place — now he could have told you,' said Amos. 'But then he left ten days ago and a new feller come in.' He turned his head and spat into

100

the darkness. 'You have had a run-a-round and no mistake. Anyway, you be 'ere now, so you'd better come on an' see Ada.'

With that, he led off across the yard and, grabbing my case, I followed closely behind.

We passed through a narrow gate into a rather lumpy pasture.

'Over 'ere,' said Amos, shining his light. The glow picked up Ada, lying full-length on her side, stomach distended and udder full and swollen, her teats dribbling milk. The breathing was heavy and irregular, otherwise she was very still. Then, the light caught her eye and momentarily she gave a weak struggle and lay still once again. Standing alongside was her calf, looking very bewildered, and as I drew closer it pushed up against its mother's body for protection.

'Don't worry, little fellow,' called Amos. 'We won't hurt you. Just goin' to make your mam better.'

'Guernsey, is she?' I asked.

'Ay,' replied Amos. 'An' he's cross Hereford from the "Bull with the Bowler Hat"!'

'"Bull with the Bowler Hat"?' I questioned. 'What's that?'

'H'artificial h'insemination,' chuckled Amos. 'I ain't got no bull.'

'When did she calve?' I bent down to examine Ada's head.

'Friday, dinner time,' he answered.

'How many has she had, Mr Breeze?'

'This'll be her third, an' you call me Amos!'

'Right, Amos,' I replied and continued my examination. Ada's muzzle was very dry and her pupils dilated. She was sweating, even though it was cold, and her coat from head to tail was damp. I drew each of her teats in turn, but the milk was good and there was no sign of clots that would indicate mastitis. Then I checked her temperature and the thermometer registered 99°F, which was one and a half degrees below normal.

'Milk fever,' I announced, as I concluded my examination.

'Thought it was,' said Amos. 'Years since I seen it, but I thought it was.'

'She's a Channel Island breed and they're particularly susceptible, due to the richness of their milk,' I commented. 'And now I would like some hot water to warm the injection.'

'Ain't you going to pump 'er?' asked Amos.

'Pump her!' I exclaimed.

'Ay, pump up the tits and tie them off.'

I smiled. 'No, we've advanced a bit since those days. Let's get the hot water and I'll tell you.'

On the way back to the house I explained to Amos how 'Milk Fever' was really an out of date term for the condition which was caused by a calcium deficiency due to the drain at calving, all the minerals going into the calf's bones and the milk supply. 'It's not a fever at all,' I told him. 'In fact the temperature drops. When calcium is short it upsets the muscle action and the cow becomes weak and collapses.'

'Well, I've seen 'em pump the udder up for it,' said Amos.

'The old idea was to try to push back the milk into the blood stream and replace the calcium,' I said, 'but it wasn't very successful. Now-a-days we inject it directly into the vein, but it's got to be blood heat and that's why I want the hot water.'

I warmed the bottle of calcium solution in the bucket that Amos provided and we returned to the paddock and poor old Ada.

With a rope around her neck to bring up the jugular vein, I prepared the flutter valve and injection equipment.

The little calf became very inquisitive, nuzzling under my arm, and Amos had to hold it back so that I could work.

'You can't have no tea for a bit,' he told the little mite. 'You just hang on.'

Taking a large needle, by the light of the tilly I chose my spot and swiftly stabbed into the vein.

'Good shot!' exclaimed Amos, as a fine stream of blood spurted out. Quickly I connected the injection apparatus, inverted the bottle and slackened the neck rope. Holding it aloft, I allowed the liquid to trickle slowly into Ada's blood stream.

It took all of five minutes, during which time Amos and I stood silently. The calf stopped struggling, Ada's breathing eased and, save for a soft gurgling in the bottle and a shivering of wind in the trees, there was no sound.

When the solution had gone I withdrew the needle from the vein.

'How long will it take?' asked Amos, letting the calf go.

'Minutes,' I replied. 'It's very rapid. We'll sit her up shortly. Shine the lamp on her nose.'

As I watched, tiny beads of moisture began to appear on Ada's dry muzzle and increased in number until her nose was quite wet.

'There!' I said, beckoning to Amos. 'It's beginning to work.'

'How can you tell that?' he said, peering over my shoulder.

'See those drops of moisture on her nose? Well, they come from little glands controlled by small muscles. Shortage of calcium stops them working, but once it's replaced, they open up and the nose becomes wet again — it's the first sign.'

The response was good and, with a bit of a heave, we got Ada sitting up.

'Don't want her to stand too quickly,' I told Amos. 'Let her take it steadily.'

As soon as Ada got her bearings, she looked around anxiously for her calf. The little chap bawled, as if to say, 'Here I am, Mum!' and struggled to her.

'I'm afraid he's not going to be able to feed for a bit,' I said. 'Otherwise, if he takes too much milk from her, she'll go down again.'

'I'll put him in a pen for tonight and give him a drop off Blossom,' Amos decided. 'She's only calved a day or so.'

'She can feed him tomorrow night, it should be all right then.' As we spoke, Ada shook herself and shakily and rather hesitantly straightened her hind legs. For a few seconds she rested on her knees, then, with a great effort, she stood upright.

'Well done, Mr Lasgarn!' said Amos. 'You've cured her!'

'It's the calcium, not me,' I replied, but I was feeling pretty pleased that Ada had not let me down. 'She'll be all right now.' And I gave the old girl a grateful pat on the rump.

Over a steaming mug of tea, Amos apologised for having to call me out at such an unearthly hour, for it was now well past three o'clock on Sunday morning.

'Did you expect her to have trouble?' I asked. 'I mean, she could have been down all night if you hadn't seen her.'

Amos bowed his head and chuckled to himself, then he looked up and smiled.

'Well, I'll tell you, Mr Lasgarn,' he said. 'You see, Saturday night I goes down to the pub. Has a few with one an' another and puts the world to rights, so you might say.' He rubbed his stubbly chin with the palm of his hand. 'Well, as I come up the lane, I looked over to Ada and 'er was staggering. Then I thought, "It could be you, me gel, an' then it could be me." So I come on in, an' sat down for an hour, an' when I went back out, 'er was still staggering — so I said, "It's you this time, my gel." An' that's when I sent for you!'

It was well past four when I finally crawled into my bed, still grinning to myself at Amos Breeze's interpretation of clinical observation.

Four

The 'small animal' consulting room in the Hacker's practice resembled an exotic plant house. It consisted of a glass-constructed lean-to, at the back of the premises, with a small waiting room accessible from the reception area, where Miss Billings reigned supreme.

A solid white-painted examination table with a linoleum top acted as centre-piece and to one side a similarly painted chest of drawers held cotton wool, bandages, plaster of paris and various requirements for the treatment of pets. A wash-hand basin was fixed to the wall and, next to the door that led into the garden, stood an oldfashioned hatstand, on which hung a single white coat. But the feature that gave this consulting room such character, and one which I had never seen in such profusion, was the collection of potted plants that adorned the shelves. There were hart's tongue ferns and geraniums, aspidistras small and large, and countless other unidentifiable creeping growths, that either hung low in knotted masses or spiralled to the roof, like hops gone mad.

Mr Hacker Senior had found great relaxation in tending his plants, and perhaps his intense involvement with animals during his working day needed such an antidote, as the soft green, slow-growing, silent, inoffensive forms provided. Miss Billings had voluntarily taken over their care and well-being, faithfully watering them and taking out the dead leaves, often with tears in her eyes.

Although the practice was mainly agricultural, it did cater for domestic pets on a regular basis, holding a surgery every evening from six o'clock until seven. The first veterinary surgeon back from farm visits attended to the clients and, during my first two weeks, it happened that I saw most of them.

Generally about four or five cases were patiently waiting, Miss Billings having already sorted them out in order of priority — based mainly on whom she liked and whom she didn't.

Dealing with these 'small animals' and their owners was a complete contrast to the farm work, where the majority of treatments were based on economics. Of course, even in pet practice, the cost of consultations and drugs still had to be taken into consideration, but I soon realised that human emotions and sentiment were very much part of the picture.

When farmers discussed the symptoms of sick animals, they did it using everyday colloquialisms, without embarrassment or hesitation. 'Straining', 'scouring', 'blowing' and 'bagging' all denoted specific conditions. But when pet owners described symptoms it was different, and often the search for the right words could take quite a time. 'How shall I put it then? Sort of a . . . well it's a . . .' Sometimes it was quite perplexing, especially when the symptoms of affected parts were related to the human, rather than the animal body — such as a large lady demonstrating on herself her bitch's swollen mammary gland, or an old gentleman describing a sore patch on his dog's left testicle.

But even in my brief encounter with the pet-owning public, I was beginning to realise the social link that animals had with humans. In the farming world dogs, cats, rabbits and cage birds were of little significance, but to the lonely, timid and unfulfilled, as well as to happy, complete and confident folk, pets were very important.

To say that people projected their own images onto their pets would have been far too sweeping a statement, but it was obvious to me, even in those early days, that a personality bond was very evident in many cases. Sometimes the personalities were so intertwined that it was difficult to tell clearly who was what!

This was my dilemma when, at my second Monday night surgery, a large red-faced man in a ragged woollen fisherman's jersey, half-mast moleskin trousers and great, odd-shaped leather boots, tugged a reluctant, sad-faced Alsatian dog into the exotic plant consulting room for my attention.

'Tom Blisset's the name,' he announced in a gruff voice, 'and this 'ere is Shaun.' The Alsatian sat down and looked away, as if trying to indicate his lack of interest in the proceedings.

'What's the problem, Mr Blisset?' I asked.

'Tom. You call me Tom!' he replied, rather threateningly.

'What's the problem, Tom?' I repeated, as the scruffy character leaned purposefully towards me.

''E's a failed guard dog,' he whispered confidentially.

At that Shaun turned round and looked up at me, as if to say, 'I heard that.'

'Stupid 'e is,' continued Tom. 'Don' know why I took 'im.' He glowered at the poor creature, who hung his head appropriately and gazed at the floor.

'Well, what can I do for you?' I enquired, thinking that the correction of failed guard dogs was more a training than a veterinary problem.

''E's got a rash on 'is belly,' explained Tom, rubbing his own ample stomach in circular motion with his hand. 'Ad it about a week. I put some goose grease on 'im, but 'e kept a-lickin' it and making 'imself sick. Stupid dog!'

Now, stupid Shaun may have been, but thick he certainly was, in the physical sense anyway. One hundred and twenty pounds of muscle and blood that would have taken a small crane to get up onto the table.

'Will he roll over on the floor?' I asked.

'ROLL OVER, SHAUN!' roared Tom, in such a deep voice that several of the plant pots rattled on the shelf.

But Shaun didn't budge, he continued to gaze at the floor.

'ROLL OVER, SHAUN!' bellowed Tom.

The only effect of the second outburst was to make a notice about Distemper Vaccination, which had been stuck to the wall with tape, slide gently to the floor.

Shaun remained immobile.

Then, to my surprise, Tom's voice rose two octaves and, bending on one knee, he softened his tone and made a plea.

'Come on, Shaun. Roll over.'

He lowered himself to both knees and went up another octave.

'Shaun. Roll over.'

With still no response from his animal, the 'Master' then laid his sixteen-stone bulk on the surgery floor, turned on his back, raised his lumpy boots in the air, so that his trousers shuffled to his knees, and made one last, valiant attempt.

'Come on, Shaun, for Christ's sake. You stupid animal!' he wheezed, his face becoming fiery red.

It was only then that Shaun moved. He raised his head slowly and looked at me. Then he looked down at the quivering body, legs waggling in the air. Then he looked back at me and his eyes said it all:

'Stupid. Who? Me? That's a laugh!'

Tom Blisset lay exhausted on his back, mumbling to himself, while Shaun and I looked on.

'Come on,' I said finally to the Alsatian. 'Roll over, please.'

Without any further bidding the dog lay down alongside his master and turned onto his right side, giving me an ample view of his affected abdomen. It was obvious that he was suffering from a mild eczema and, as he lay quite still, I was able to make an adequate examination of the condition.

'You can both get up now,' I said, when I had finished.

Tom, with considerable puffing and blowing, eventually

regained a standing position after three attempts, but Shaun still lay recumbent.

'GET UP, SHAUN!' he hollered.

There was no response.

'Blast, if 'e won't use 'is legs now!' said Tom, shaking his head in disbelief.

'Get up, Shaun, please,' I said.

And Shaun got to his feet.

Tom eyed me suspiciously.

'It's probably due to his feeding,' I commented. 'Eruptions of the skin often occur if it's not balanced.'

'Butcher's offal, I gives 'im,' said Tom, still looking at me thoughtfully.

'Could be a bit rich. Some biscuits or biscuit meal would be advisable, to cut down on the protein.'

'I'll get some,' said Tom.

'And I'll give you some tablets to ease the irritation. It should clear in a week or so.'

He never said another word as I counted out the tablets and wrote down the instructions on the packet, nor when he paid his fee. He just mumbled a 'Goodbye' when he opened the door.

'Come on, Shaun,' he said.

But the dog did not move.

'Please!' added Tom, glaring at me as he did so.

And with that, Shaun gave a deft wag of his tail and followed obediently.

There followed two fairly straightforward cases, one of a dog with inflamed ears and another a sneezing cat, and then Miss Billings came through and shut the door behind her.

'All finished?' I asked, as she folded her arms and inflated her woolly jumper.

'Just that woman!' she said disdainfully.

'That woman?' I questioned, slightly mystified.

'Calls herself Miss Lafont.' Miss Billings' face began to colour. 'Pretends she's French. Huh! She's no more French than my Aunt Fanny!'

I sensed a slight degree of antagonism in the air and decided to tread carefully, but Miss Billings was in full flow: 'She said she only wants to see Mr McBean. I told her he wouldn't be coming back this evening. Of course, he plays up to her, the hussie, and she flaps those big artificial eyelashes of hers — quite a pantomime, I can tell you!'

I had never seen Miss Billings in this state before and was quite keen to view the subject of her malevolence.

'But Mr McBean *isn't* coming back this evening,' I confirmed. 'So what is she going to do?'

'After a highly dramatic performance in the waiting room, Her Ladyship has decided that Petal is in distress, so she will see you!'

'Oh!' I said, trying to subdue my obvious interest. Whether the fact that I rubbed my hands together, in the manner of C. J. Pink, gave my thoughts away, I wasn't sure, but Miss Billings shot me a look of absolute contempt. 'Men!' she said in exasperation and left, slamming the door behind her.

I cleaned the table, straightened my tie and waited in anticipation for Miss Lafont. Even before she came in, I was conscious of her perfume and, when she did appear, she was just as I might have imagined — slim, attractive, dark haired and sexily dressed. She wore a white, low-cut frilly blouse, with a rose nestling cheekily in the centre, black skirt with a tempting slit up one side and very high-heeled white shoes. She floated towards me with Petal under her arm. Petal was a French Poodle, also slim and attractive as poodles go, blondish and sporting a jewelled collar, and if Miss Billings was to be believed, was probably short on French blood as well.

Miss Lafont came to a halt by the examination table, but her perfume travelled on, lulling me into a state of mind that I only just managed to crop in the nick of time.

'What can I do for you both?' I cooed.

She giggled, squeezed Petal closely to her ample bosom and said: 'Who's been a naughty girl, then? Who's been a

110

fast little madam?' I detected a slight Birminghamese in her Gallic accent, but as far as I was concerned it was a minor flaw. Petal reacted with a couple of barks, which had no French accent at all.

'We went out when we shouldn't,' Miss Lafont continued, laughing, 'and we did things that we shouldn't.' She looked at me and fluttered her eyelashes. Artificial they may have been, but they worked a treat. 'We're naughty, aren't we!' she said smiling and, without taking her eyes off me, kissed Petal upon her nose.

'What a naughty girl,' I said, entering into the spirit of things. 'Petal, I am surprised at you.' I winked at the little poodle, but Miss Lafont took my gesture personally and patted the air between us coyly with a heavily-jewelled hand. 'When did it happen?' I asked.

'Last night, after supper. Down in Bishop's Meadow.' she shook her head knowingly at Petal and then turned again to me. 'Perhaps I should have rung you then. You wouldn't have minded, would you?' she asked, slipping her eyelashes into top gear.

'Of course not,' I gushed. 'It would be no trouble, any time. But don't you worry, Miss Lafont...'

'Mimi,' she said. 'You can call me Mimi.' After being asked to address Tom Blisset as 'Tom' and now Miss Lafont as 'Mimi', I thought to myself what a sociable lot the Hackers' clients were. Taking a deep breath I continued:

'Don't you worry, Mimi.' I paused and she nodded approvingly. 'Everything will be all right. Just one little injection and her problems will be over.'

'Oh! Isn't that wonderful, Petal? Just one teensy-weensy injection.'

She smiled appreciatively and I turned away to the chest of drawers. My hand was on the bottle of oestrogen-based injection, when Miss Lafont added: 'This injection must be new. How marvellous. Last time she had a hay seed in her ear, Mr McBean had a terrible job getting it out!'

I stood with my back to them, remembering Pink's Law: 'Never make a diagnosis on one factor alone.' Even if it was as delicious as Mimi Lafont. My hand strayed over to the auroscope.

'We'd better have a look at it first,' I said, recovering my composure, and as I investigated Petal's ear canal, I thought what a fool I had nearly made myself look. There was no sign of a hay seed of any description; in fact, come to think of it, it was quite unlikely at that time of year.

'Well, she was shaking her head a bit,' said Mimi Lafont, demurely.

'Possibly a slight inflamation, some ear drops should soothe it,' I advised.

'You are sure?' she asked.

'Yes,' I replied, as firmly as I was capable.

'Do you think I should bring Petal back, just to be safe?' she suggested, smiling sweetly.

'Certainly,' I agreed. 'How about Friday?'

'We'd love to come on Friday,' she said.

I gently ran some drops into Petal's left ear. 'I'll do the right one as well, just to balance things up,' I explained.

'Doesn't he think of everything!' Mimi Lafont purred. 'We haven't seen you before. What's your name?'

'Hugh Lasgarn.' I attempted to make it as interesting as I could.

'How nice,' she said. 'Sounds quite foreign.'

'Welsh,' I explained.

'Welsh!' she laughed. 'How different.'

Not knowing quite how to take her reaction, I said: 'Mr McBean will probably be able to see you on Friday, if you wish.'

She gasped, then breathed in deeply and inflated the white blouse in a way that Miss Billings, in her wildest dreams, would have been unable to match.

'Oh! We'd like to see *you* again, wouldn't we, darling?' And with that, she thrust Petal forward and the poodle licked my face vigorously.

'She likes you,' said Mimi dreamily. 'See you on Friday.'

And sweeping her pet back into her arms, she left. But her perfume lingered on.

I tidied up the chest of drawers and put the Distemper notice back upon the wall. As I passed through reception, I called 'Goodnight' to Miss Billings. But she didn't answer.

*   *   *

'Market inspection for you,' said Bob Hacker, two days later. 'We do it on behalf of the Council. Nothing too strenuous, just a general appraisal of the stock for contagious diseases, severe lameness, ringworm, that sort of thing. If you see any animal in very poor condition you have the authority to forbid sale, and in extreme cases prosecute. There's an RSPCA Inspector and a Policeman on duty, so if you have a problem of that nature, get in touch with them.'

'Is that likely?' I asked.

'No,' said Bob, 'Ledingford Market has a pretty good standard on the whole, but there are occasional lapses. Quite a few dealers do business there and some of those want watching. The drovers are generally careful, but if you should see anyone mistreating or abusing an animal, then jump in and stop it and report the chap to the Market Superintendent. The only other problem you are likely to get is a dispute, when the auctioneers will call on you to arbitrate. Be careful, because there are tricks of the trade and the lads down there know them all.'

The market was situated in the centre of the town and was buzzing with activity when I drove through the gates. It appeared to be absolute chaos, with stock wagons, cars, people and animals all going in different directions. Right ahead of me were the sheep pens, packed with woolly bodies and surrounded by a crowd, who seemed hypnotised by the white-coated auctioneer, standing quite perilously on a gang plank that ran along the top of the rails.

My progress was very much a stop-go procedure, for every few yards I was halted by small clutches of farmers, either in earnest conversation or slapping each other's backs and roaring with laughter. Nobody moved with any great degree of urgency and, as I eased the little Ford through the crowd, I virtually had to shove some of them gently to one side.

Bob Hacker had said that there was a reserved space for the vet by the Market Office, a low bricked building near the cattle ring. As I made my way towards it I felt quite enlivened by my newly acquired position of authority as Market Inspector, and to have a reserved space for my car did my ego a power of good.

In fact, as I rounded the building I was confronted with a row of cars, each parked facing named signs, such as Market Superintendent, Auctioneer, Council Inspector, and at the end, Veterinary Surgeon. The sign was bright and bold and looked very imposing; there was only one thing wrong: there was no space. Where my car was due to park stood a dilapidated red van, its wing loose and rusted, the side windows cracked and partly boarded up and rear door handles and number plate secured by string. It looked highly unlikely that it belonged to another vet, so I decided to investigate. As I peered through the crack in the rear doors I was deafened by a ferocious barking from within. Suddenly there came a loud bang and the doors were forced partly outwards, but the string on the handle fortunately held; then a black muzzle poked through the gap and a vicious snarl revealed some very sharp teeth.

I walked to the front of the van and, like lightning, a black and white collie dog pounced on to the remnants of the front seat and gave a most aggressive display of possession. The dog leaped up and down in a frenzy and, as I watched the little van rock from side to side a voice behind me shouted, 'You can't park there!' I turned to find a very portly policeman bearing down upon me.

'You can't park there, you will have to move,' he said.

'Well, I should be able to park there,' I replied, pointing to the red van, 'I'm the vet.'

'The vet?' he queried.

'Hugh Lasgarn,' I said, holding out my hand, 'I'm with

Mr Hacker.'

'Oh yes! Sorry about the old gentleman.' He held out his hand in return. 'Bob Packham!' The policeman studied the red van for a moment, then turned to me and said:

'Sam Juggins!'

'His van?' I asked.

'It is,' replied PC Packham. 'So that's where he put it. Come up to me a few minutes ago and said, 'If my vehicle is in the way, officer, you can move it.' He smiled and shook his head. 'Bit of a rogue is Sam, but he ain't all bad. You move it, Mr Lasgarn, and put your car in.'

'Move it?' I said incredulously.

'Ay,' he replied. 'Stick it over there, by that wall.'

I banged the van with my fist and all hell was let loose inside.

'You move it, Constable,' I said, the ferocious barking nearly drowning my words.

PC Packham, hands on hips, squinted through the crack in the door and stepped back sharply as the collie's teeth appeared.

'I'll 'ave 'is guts for garters!' he exploded. 'Move it be damned. You stick yours by that wall and I'll go and find 'im,' and he trudged off to apprehend the culprit.

I parked by the opposite wall and set off on my tour of inspection.

The market was a fascinating place, and it was obviously as much a social occasion as it was a general sale. There were at least three hundred people milling about amongst the stock, most of them farmers and every one so different. Physically there was a tremendous variation, from the accustomed type of jovial, portly, ruddy-complexioned man, to some who were tall and pale, and others so bent it was difficult to see their features at all.

But, whether Welsh or English, each and every one was involved in the gathering in a purposeful way. If not talking, dealing, bidding or driving stock, they were looking over pens of ewes or bunches of bullocks, pressing down through the curly fleeces to tell the bodily condition, or pinching the flanks of store cattle to estimate their firmness.

I passed through the pig section where great hairy sows, with countless pink piglets scurrying about their feet, were for sale, and watched with interest as bunches of porkers, squealing hysterically, were expertly directed down alleyways and into pens by drovers with large flat boards.

In the poultry shed, a completely different atmosphere prevailed, and the vendors and purchasers were also of a different nature. In fact, at first glance, they even appeared bird-like themselves — the men with beaky noses and the women puffed up and rounded, like some of the fat old hens in the cages. Bantams and geese, long-necked ducks and a colourful array of poultry, all changing hands amid a cacophony of clucking, squawking and high-pitched talking.

The quality of stock was good, and I could see that there were no signs of overcrowding of the pens, or ill-treatment of any sort.

I was standing listening to the banter of the auctioneer at the sheep pens, when the loudspeaker crackled out a message.

'Will the Veterinary Surgeon please go to the cattle ring, the Veterinary Surgeon please to the cattle ring, immediately!'

My heart began to beat just a little faster. 'To the cattle ring, immediately!'

It was the urgency of the call that disturbed me, and I hurriedly made my way over to the far side of the market.

The ring had not long been erected, in memory of a local worthy. It was of brick construction and was situated at the end of the covered pens. There was tiered seating for a few hundred, looking down upon the railed sale ring, at the back of which stood the auctioneer's booth.

As I approached I could hear the steady monotones of the auctioneer's voice, as he controlled the bidding. The sound allayed one of my fears: that an animal had collapsed and I might be called to attend to it before a

116

considerable gallery.

Making my way through the crowd gathered by the ring, I reached the steps of the rostrum. There were several people in the box as well as the auctioneer, a tall impressive man with a tweed cap and long grey sideboards. As he rattled out the bids on a large red shorthorn cow, his assistants, like hawks, scoured the gathering for nods, winks, coughs and minuscule gestures indicating an offer. For the life of me I couldn't see any significant movement, but the money kept rising all the time.

A young man in a pork pie hat looked round at me.

'Vet,' I said.

'Ah, yes.' He took me by the arm and led me around the corner, beyond the range of the verbal barrage.

'Peter Shackleton,' he said. 'Part of Shackleton & Co. You're new, aren't you?'

'Yes. Hugh Lasgarn.'

'With Hacker's?'

'Yes, for a short while.'

Young Shackleton looked about him rather nervously, then said, 'Bit of a sticky one and we'd like your opinion. Someone's chucked up one of Denthall's cows!'

When I made no comment he looked at me rather strangely, then he snapped his finger.

'Of course, Denthall wouldn't mean a thing to you.'

I shook my head. 'Never heard of him.'

'You will do if you are here long enough,' Shackleton replied. 'Brings about twenty cows a week, does a lot of business here, very important man.' He looked at me directly, his eyes reiterating his last sentence.

'What's the reason?' I asked.

'Chap who's bought it says it's got mastitis and we'd like you to arbitrate. She's in the lairage, I'll take you over.'

The lairage was a long shed running parallel to the covered pens, housing fresh-calved dairy cows, before and after their appearance in the adjacent sale ring. Friesians, Shorthorns, Ayrshires, all brushed up and in show condition, were tied in stalls, but there was no doubt where the attention was centred, for at the end of the shed a small crowd had gathered, buzzing with conversation.

Peter Shackleton pushed through and I followed. In the stall stood a good-looking Friesian cow, her coat shining, her tail brushed and fanned out elegantly behind her. Hooves and horns sparkled and the udder that expanded between her legs looked full and silky. She really was a picture.

'This is Mr Parry, who's just bought her,' said Shackleton. 'He says she's wrong.'

Mr Parry was a small man, his face pale and drawn and his appearance in no way enhanced by the crumpled black suit he wore. His shirt and tie, too, were creased and he squeezed his well-worn hands together nervously.

'She's got a hard quarter,' he said. 'I think she's had mastitis.'

'Didn't you examine her before you bid?' I asked.

'Wouldn't give me no proper chance,' he replied.

'Don't want everybody poking at 'em!' said a swarthy individual in a brown coat. 'Anyway, I didn't think he was looking to buy.' He looked rather contemptuously at the little man.

'Mr Denthall's cowman,' said Shackleton, motioning to the man in the brown coat.

The crowd had increased in size and I sensed the air of anticipation behind me. 'We'd like you to arbitrate,' said Shackleton. 'Just to see that she's all right.' He nodded and gave a weak smile.

'Of course she's all right!' The crowd parted and a large arrogant figure, in a stetson-type trilby and camel coat, walked forward. His face was full-coloured and podgy, his eyes small but very blue, and in his teeth he gripped a half-smoked Havana.

'There's nowt wrong with that cow,' he said, thrusting his left hand deeply into his expensive coat pocket. 'She's right and straight. I don't bring rubbish to this market, and Shackleton here knows that well!'

Peter Shackleton shuffled uneasily.

'Mr Parry says she's got a hard quarter,' I said.

'Rubbish!' shouted Denthall. 'Natural wedging after calving, any fool can see that. Paid more than he wanted to, that's the real trouble. Well, I'll not have that; sold under the hammer she was and that's it!' He chewed aggressively on his cigar.

'I can afford it,' said Mr Parry. 'But I don't want a three-quartered cow!'

'This is Mr Lasgarn, the vet,' said Shackleton. 'He's going to arbitrate.'

Denthall turned aside and glowered at me, his tiny eyes cold and hostile, then suddenly his manner altered, and a calculated smile developed on his face.

'Oh well!' he exclaimed. 'The vet, eh!' He placed a large fat hand on my shoulder. 'Well, let's see what the young gentleman thinks, then. See if he can tell the difference between a normal bagging and mastitis.' He turned and surveyed the attendant crowd and nodded knowingly. Shackleton stood back. The man in the brown coat held the tail to one side.

'Try her and see,' said Denthall, in a syrupy tone.

I ran my hand over the upper part of the udder, feeling for enlarged glands, but none were obvious. The skin was taut and, beneath, the tissue was full and doughy, indicating post-calving swelling. But, as Denthall had said, that was normal. To the left back quarter I gave special attention. Although its consistency was very similar it did feel slightly larger, but not a great deal. I drew the milk from the other three quarters — it was creamy, with no clots or lumps — and then I drew the milk from the left back quarter.

'How's that, vet?' It was Denthall peering over my shoulder.

'It appears all right,' I agreed.

'There,' he shouted triumphantly. 'What did I tell you! I never bring no rubbish to market.'

I stood back and studied the cow. Mr Parry studied my

face, but said nothing. I tried not to look at him, but I could feel his sad, appealing eyes burning into my cheek.

The quarter *was* slightly larger, but it was difficult to be sure. The milk appearance was normal, and yet I felt that I was giving in to Denthall's pressure; but I couldn't hedge, I had to make a decision.

Denthall, Parry, Shackleton and a couple of dozen faces awaited my pronouncement.

I was just about to speak when I felt a nudge in my ribs and then came a hoarse whisper from behind: 'Strip it out!' I half turned, but the stocky figure behind me turned away, too. I just caught a glimpse of a red neck-a-chief protruding from an ill-fitting tweed jacket. The adviser, if that was him, pulled the peak of his cap down slightly, as if to retain his anonymity.

As I turned back, he must have turned too, for again came the whispered instruction: 'Get him to strip it out!' I got the message, and sound advice it was too; if that was done it would make a diagnosis a hundred times easier.

'I'd like it stripped out,' I said. The effect of my request was quite momentous. Shackleton looked up like a startled rabbit, little Mr Parry put his hand to his lips and bit his finger. Denthall seemed ready to explode and the crowd remained in an uneasy silence. Then Denthall did explode, quite violently.

'Strip 'er out! Strip 'er out!' he raged. 'Can't you bloody well tell? There's nowt wrong, any fool could tell that without stripping her out!'

'Maybe,' I said, as calmly as I could. 'But to make a reasonable diagnosis I want her milked.'

'I'll take 'er home first!' stormed Denthall.

'You can't do that,' chipped in little Mr Parry. 'She was knocked down to me, so I've got the choice. Get your chap to strip her out.'

The brown coated man looked at Denthall, who in turn took a hasty look at the crowd around.

'Go on, strip her out!' shouted a voice from the back.

'Yes, go on,' said a few others.

Realising his position, Denthall nodded.

The man in the brown coat certainly could milk and, urged on by the contagious anger of his boss, powered the streams of milk into the bucket, so that it frothed up spectacularly.

'I'll have a word with your father about this,' Denthall threatened, glaring at young Shackleton. 'If you can't take my word, I'll not come here any more. There's other markets and auctioneers as good as this!' But Shackleton said nothing.

Finally, after half filling a second bucket, the brown coated man dragged his stool away. I stepped forward and gently examined the left hind quarter. As I probed into the now slack substance, my fingers came across three hard lumps, two plum-size and one a little larger, evidence of damage caused by previous mastitis. The other quarters were clear.

I stood up and looked Denthall straight in his piggy blue eyes.

'Chronic mastitis,' I said. 'Mr Parry is right.'

Denthall seethed on the spot, then, taking the butt end of his cigar from his mouth, flung it to the floor. 'Bloody vets!' he roared and charged away.

A satisfied murmur ran through the crowd and they started to disperse. 'Thank you, vet.' It was Mr Parry. 'Thank you for standing up for me.'

I nodded and we shook hands. Poor Mr Parry, he didn't know how close it had been.

'Thanks,' said Peter Shackleton. 'I'd better go and report to Father.'

I looked about for the red neck-a-chief, but the people had already moved on and he was nowhere to be seen.

I spent the rest of my inspection walking about in a slight daze. The incident had taken all my energy, although one or two folks did smile and say 'Hello', and I realised that my performance must have made some impact.

At half past twelve I reported to the Market Superintendent's office, as Bob Hacker had told me.

'All in order,' I advised him through the wooden hatch.

'Turned down one of Mr Denthall's cows, I hear,' he said, looking over his glasses.

I nodded.

'Well, well,' he replied. 'Well, well.'

With mixed feelings I went back to the car. As I approached the parking spot, I noticed the red van still in my place. The back doors were now open and a pair of stocky buttocks protruded from them. The owner was wrestling with a white-faced calf. I could hear the collie dog yelping on the front seat and its presence triggered off my annoyance. A few sharp words were in order, I thought.

'You've got no right to park here, this is the vet's spot,' I told the buttocks firmly.

There was a puffing and blowing as the body withdrew and straightened up.

'You mustn't park here,' I repeated. 'It's for vets.'

'And you be the vet, be you?' came the reply, as the man turned round and grinned broadly. 'Pleased to meet you.' He held out a hand. 'I'm Sam Juggins.'

And it was then that my eye caught sight of the red neck-a-chief tied at his throat.

*   *   *

The market incident had unsettled me and I was glad to be able to chat things over with McBean at the end of the day. I found our evening meetings in the Hopman both relaxing and reassuring and a great help to my confidence, which was still rather shaky.

Well, now! You were truly blooded on your first inspection, Hugh. But it'll not do you any harm,' commented McBean wryly, after I had recounted my confrontation with Denthall. 'He's a nasty piece of work at any time and I've had more than one barney with the devil, myself.'

'It was Sam Juggins who saved me,' I admitted.

122

'Now, isn't that life!' said McBean, smoothing down his moustache. 'To a lot of people, Sam is a rogue and Denthall a lord, but Sam's an honest rogue, if you know what I mean. He may bend the rules a bit, but he'll never leave anyone in trouble.'

I went to the bar and bought another round.

'Met a rather special client of yours, last night,' I said to McBean, as I set the full tankards back on the table.

He raised his bushy eyebrows. 'Now who might that be?' he enquired.

'Mimi Lafont.'

'And Petal,' he added, a mischievous grin creeping over his face. 'Not another hay seed?'

'How did you guess?' I answered.

'She comes fairly regularly, ever since I removed one in the Summer. Just for a bit of a check, you know. And what did you diagnose, yourself?'

'First of all, I took the wrong track,' I admitted. Then I told McBean how I had erroneously concluded from her description, that Petal had been the unfortunate victim of some lusty, canine Casanova in the Bishop's Meadow. 'I was just going to give the stilboestrol, when she mentioned hayseeds,' I explained.

McBean burst into laughter. 'Well, Hugh! That's surely one of the best,' he exclaimed, wiping his eyes.

'You certainly added two and two into five there, my boy.'

'She's coming again on Friday,' I added.

McBean ceased his laughter. 'Is she, now?' he said, suspiciously. 'Well, Hugh, lad. We'll have to see you don't get led astray.'

'Why?' I asked 'Could be good experience for a young vet.'

'Time yet,' replied McBean.

'But I've only got thirty days, less than that now,' I reminded him. 'Anyway, you should talk. Five years qualified and not even courting.'

McBean grasped the handle of his pint and raised it

before his eyes, studying the clear amber brew intently, as if examining it for certification.

'I'll get married when I'm good and ready,' he said, without averting his gaze. 'I'm good enough now — but I'm not yet ready.'

Then he set into his pint and lowered it in one go.

Five

Charlie had described Wales as 'lumpy' and in many respects his description was apt. Once south-west of the River Wye, the flat water meadows receded and the countryside became ridged, forming three valleys running west to south-east. The first and most fertile was the Golden Valley, which opened out into plains of arable farmland. Next and much narrower came Lindenchurch where, although the land appeared rich, the living was just a shade harder. The fields tended to be smaller, the trees more round-shouldered, the hedges tighter and the farm buildings strategically sited to avoid the wicked Welsh winds.

But it was the last valley, the Shepwall, that left the most lasting impression upon all who visited it. Steepsided from the north, the fields covering the lower slopes formed small neat squares, yet the farmsteads were few and isolated. The south side, however, displayed the grandest feature. Wild and beautiful, it rose through bracken and gorse, two thousand feet and more. A sombre wall whose top, often masked by threatening cloud, took the full force of the rain-bearing south-westerlies. Storms could lash the rocky steps and shelves, whilst down below the valley basked in sunshine.

How fittingly named, that brooding barrier to 'lumpy' Wales: the Black Mountain.

It was on the Friday morning of my second week that I was to discover the Shepwall valley.

I had been given two calls. The first and most urgent was to a Mrs Sarah Williams of Pontavon Farm where, during the night, a calf had died and others in the bunch were unwell. Mrs Williams was a widow with a young family, her husband having succumbed the previous year to a massive heart attack.

'Worked himself into an early grave,' McBean had commented when he gave me the instructions. 'Good woman, lovely family, very, very sad. She didn't give much history about the calves, it could be blackleg or even acute pneumonia. Anyway, Hugh, get there as soon as you can, she's rather upset about it all. Then, when you've finished, go back up the valley to Howell Powell. Mrs Williams will give you directions.'

Howell Powell apparently had a lame cow that needed attention. According to McBean, he was an odd character, treating most animal ailments with his own personal remedies.

'Don't suppose we go there more than twice a year,' McBean had added as he further studied the ledger lying on the sacred counter. 'And when you've done, give a ring back from Evan's shop at St Madoc's. You can use his telephone, but remember, he'll listen to everything you say. And don't forget to pay for the call.'

I took on petrol from the handcranked pump in the yard and topped up the radiator which had developed a slight leak, then checked that I had all my equipment.

The late G. R. Hacker had devised a veterinary box that rode on the back seat of the car and was of sturdy wooden construction, not unlike a small cabin trunk. The interior was divided into compartments that accommodated bottles of medicine, tins of tablets and packets of powders from which cattle drenches were prepared. In the boot there was a metal box containing all the requirements for calving cows, such as thick and thin ropes, short sticks to use as handles and eye hooks to control movement of the head. There were also embryotome wires and guarded knives for the grisly task of dismembering dead calves that proved too difficult to deliver normally. The remainder of the tools comprised a brass stirrup pump to irrigate unclean wombs with antiseptic; a probang, a large, long and rather unwieldy leather-bound tube which, when inserted into the throat, could unblock an obstructed gullet or let out wind from an over-inflated gut; a pair of 'barnacles' — metal nose tongs to restrain a fractious patient — and a strong rope halter.

The protective clothing was minimal, and stripping to the waist for dirty jobs was the order of the day. Wellington boots and a red rubber apron were provided for messy encounters, but these could be supplemented according to personal taste. A cold rubber apron on a bare chest in the frosty air could be an enlivening experience and even the acclimatised personnel had taken steps to ease the shock.

Bob Hacker had a little sheepskin waistcoat that he wore beneath his red apron, but it was McBean, with his usual Irish ingenuity, who had developed an odd, but very practical regalia. It consisted of one of a number of old flannel shirts with the sleeves removed, which were sent to him regularly in batches from an old uncle in Connemara. To prevent any distasteful matter reaching his uncle's shirts he was equipped with what appeared to be rubber washers, circles of thin rubber cut from old car inner tubes. These he wore around his biceps, the whole weird ensemble giving him the appearance of being prepared for initiation into a secret society.

'A wee idea I picked up when I was a student working at Dublin Docks,' he confided. 'You'll see similar designs on ships' hawsers to prevent rats reaching the decks. Really ought to patent the idea, Hugh,' he said, when he proudly presented me with a pair of his creations. 'McBean's "Mucklets" could make me a fortune!'

My medical bag was similar to that of the late G. R. Hacker, which I had been privileged to use on my first case, but much more battered. However, it served its purpose and in the drawers I kept glass syringes, a ther-

127

mometer, stethoscope, small drugs and a few instruments.

Finally, having found everything in place and functional, I started on my way.

The barometric pressure had fallen and the weather had changed from bright days with frosty mornings to a milder atmosphere that caused leaden clouds to hang low over the county. Occasionally a shaft of sunlight broke through the uneasy sky, like a spotlight on a stage, and through the gap, white fluffy banks of cumulus gave a heavenly impression of the universe beyond. But as I drove west, I could see in the distance ahead that the sky was lowering to join the Black Mountain summit, erasing the horizon in a continuous lack-lustre mist.

Turning from the Gradonchurch road, I came to Colestone, a small hamlet caught in one of the spots of sunshine. The lath and plaster panels of the Tudor cottages shone brightly in the brilliant rays, accentuating the black timbers in sharp relief. Each dwelling, unique in design, reflected the ancient craftsman's art and whim. I tried to picture the industrious scene as they were built. Men digging and hauling, sawing and hammering, working with natural materials and using their hands with great satisfaction.

Woodwork was never my strongpoint. I remembered how, at school, I made an egg-holder — a simple structure consisting of a small square of wood in which I bored four holes and mounted it on a triangular plinth. I took it home to Mother, very proud of my achievement, and begged her to give me some eggs, very scarce in those days, to put into my egg-holder. But I had made the holes too large, and when I put the eggs in, they fell to the floor and smashed.

That was the last time I ever made anything in wood.

Through Colestone to Lindenchurch, past Evan's shop at St Madoc's — also known as 'Top Shop' because of its situation on the ridge overlooking the next valley. Away to my left, the shadowy outline of Capley Court was just visible through the trees, a grand and somewhat mysterious-looking mansion presenting an incongruous sight amid the wild countryside.

Two miles on and I was descending sharply to Shepwall, and halfway down the valley I came to Pontavon Farm.

Clearly visible from the road, it was more of a smallholding than a farm. A compact low-walled garden fronted a whitewashed cottage, whose single chimney merrily belched clouds of grey smoke. From the garden, a gate led onto the yard which was bordered by a cowhouse, barn, two small cots and a lean-to log shed.

Access to Pontavon was by no means straightforward, however, for between it and the road ran a small river, full and boisterous. There was a ford for vehicles and a rather willowy bridge for pedestrians. I decided it was too much to expect amphibious qualities of my gallant little car, so I elected to cross by the bridge. It creaked beneath my weight, but did not rock or sway, and I negotiated it without mishap to be greeted on the far side by two collie dogs, one excitedly barking and the other, obviously older, standing by the garden gate, wagging its tail. As they followed me I heard the sound of children's voices through the partly open cottage door. I gave three sharp knocks and the chatter ceased abruptly. I waited a while, then around the door, below latch level, appeared a small tousled head and two large brown eyes. I smiled, but before I could say a word the head was followed by another, just above it, and another pair of equally large brown eyes.

'Hullo,' I said. 'Who are you?'

My question was answered with giggles and the little girls disappeared. As they did, the door was opened wider by a young woman, Mrs Sarah Williams. She was very slender, with long dark hair hanging loosely about her shoulders. Her face was quite serene, yet seemed to mirror an inner sadness. She held up two floury hands and smiled and as she did, for a fleeting moment, a bright sparkle lit her eyes.

'I've been baking,' she said, and a trifle nervously

brushed some loose strands of hair from her forehead, leaving specks of flour on her cheek.

By now, the two small girls had reappeared, hanging on their mother's apron.

'Have you come to see Tommy's baby calf?' asked the elder girl.

'It's gone to sleep,' said the little one, sadly.

'Hugh Lasgarn. I'm with Mr Hacker,' I explained. 'And yes,' I said to the little girls, 'I have come to see the calves.'

'It was a dreadful shock and so upsetting for Tommy,' said Mrs Williams. 'He looks after them and tries so hard. He even made the feeding trough himself,' she added, proudly. 'My husband died last year, you know.' She pulled the girls closer to her.

'I'm sorry,' I said, inadequately.

'Tommy's the man of the house now,' she continued. She looked beyond me, raising her head as gracefully as a ballerina. Mrs Sarah Williams was indeed a very beautiful woman. 'Here's Tommy now, he'll tell you.'

I turned to see a curly headed boy running across the yard, his face flushed and eager as he swung through the gate.

'I saw you come,' he said breathlessly. 'I was in the top field with the sheep, so I ran back.' It was Tommy Williams, the man of the house and all of ten years old. 'They're in the cot. Come with me and I'll show you.'

As we crossed the yard, he told me how his uncle had bought six Hereford Cross calves at Abergavenny market. 'I was going to rear them up and sell them as stores in the Autumn,' he said in serious tone. 'They could be turned out in the Spring, we've got good grass at Pontavon.' Tommy chatted on, taking slightly longer strides than most ten-year-olds and conversing in rather an old-fashioned manner, probably as his father had done. A lump came to my throat as I followed him — a boy trying to do a man's job.

He didn't appear to show any remorse when he pulled back the sack on the dead calf, but I knew he was fighting tears.

'Found him dead this morning,' he said, in a matter-of-fact way. 'Took his feed like a good 'un last night.'

'Let's have a look at the rest of them,' I suggested.

'They look OK,' Tommy commented, opening the door of the calf cot. It was well strawed and clean; some sweet-smelling hay hung from a net and a long wooden trough containing the remnants of barley meal stood along the far wall.

'Made that yourself?' I asked.

'Yes,' he replied, nodding his head. 'It was an old door that Dad cut up before he . . .' Tommy turned away and I took an exaggerated step forward to examine the calves. They were in good condition; one or two seemed slightly nervous, but their eyes were bright, noses clean and coats sleek. I questioned Tommy about the feeding, watering and bedding he used.

'I think we'll open up the dead one,' I said finally. 'Do a post-mortem examination. Can you get me a bucket of water?'

'I'll only be a minute,' he said and sped off to the cottage.

Tommy paid great attention to the examination of the calf's organs as I explained the various parts and their functions to him. When I come to the heart, he knelt down beside me and studied it closely.

'What does it look like when a heart makes an attack?' he asked.

'Attack?'

'Yes, like Dad had,' he replied, looking up. 'Last year.'

They never told me about this at university. About how, one morning, I would find myself in a wild Border valley, the sound of rushing water at my back, the air still and thundery and the Black Mountain brooding silently overhead. How I would be holding a bloodstained calf's heart in my hands and, kneeling down beside me, a small boy, earnestly wanting to know how his father had died.

He was waiting for my answer.

'Rather like this one,' I told him eventually. 'Just still,

131

just very, very still.'

Then I continued the rest of my examination in silence.

There were no abnormal symptoms, apart from a few small areas in the lung, showing evidence of slight damage probably caused by a pneumonia virus, but in no way sufficient to cause death. It was when I examined the stomach contents that I found a clue. Lying in the mix of digested hay and barley meal were small black flakes, like bits of rust. I collected several and washed them carefully in the water. The lad watched closely.

'Bring me a sample of the meal, Tommy.' He leaped up and ran to another shed. But the meal he brought was fresh and pure, there were no black flakes to be seen.

I washed up and went back to the calf cot where the calves looked up inquisitively. With a clap of my hands, I startled them, causing three to move back from the door, the fourth to stand and shiver, but the fifth ran straight into the wall and banged its head. I went in and caught the last calf and waved my hand before its eyes, but it made no reaction — it was blind.

Dead calf, nervous calf, blind calf. Black flakes in the stomach. It had to be paint, lead paint. The calves were suffering from lead poisoning.

But where could they be licking paint?

Then my eyes fell on the trough that ran alongside the wall. The wooden one that Tommy had made.

I got the little lad to fetch his mother. Then I explained what had happened.

'The paint on the old door contained lead — most old paints do. The calves have been licking the trough as they were feeding and have swallowed the poisonous flakes. They are very toxic, causing nervous symptoms, blindness and death.'

Mrs Williams put her hands on her son's shoulder.

'You weren't to know, Tommy dear,' she comforted. 'It's not your fault.'

Tommy Williams put his hand to his mouth and bit his finger hard, then suddenly he started to shake and burst into tears.

'Don't be upset, Tommy.' But as I held out my hand towards him, he broke away from his mother and ran across the yard and out into the field.

The girls went to run after him, but their mother called them back. Only the dogs followed, the young one swiftly, the older one at a slower pace.

'He's best left, at the moment,' she said, understandingly. 'Best left alone. Will we lose any more, Mr Lasgarn?'

'Once nervous symptoms develop, it's not good,' I admitted. 'You could lose two more. I'll drench them all with Epsom Salts, that will combine with any free lead in the stomach and neutralise it. If it's already absorbed, then it will be more difficult to control, but I have some injections I can try.'

Mrs Williams held the calves for their treatment and when I had finished, I carried the trough into the yard.

'You could scrape the paint off, but it would never be really safe. I think it would be best to burn it,' I suggested. 'I'll come over tomorrow and check them again.'

'That's very kind, Mr Lasgarn,' she said. 'Would you like a cup of tea? I've just made some Welsh cakes. Do you like them?'

'My favourite,' I replied.

Over tea and Welsh cakes, she told me how they had come down from Breconshire and bought Pontavon, and how her husband had done ploughing and hedging for neighbouring farmers to pay for it, as well as tending to his own stock and crops.

'His ambition was to grow acres of potatoes in the Valley. They all said it wouldn't work, but he would have made it, I'm sure. He was that sort of man,' she said proudly. 'Perhaps one day Tommy will show them.' There was no self-pity in her attitude and, if there was sadness, it was more than countered by determination of spirit.

'I'm sure he will,' I agreed. 'I'm sure he will.'

I thanked her for the tea and she gave me a bag of Welsh cakes.

Tommy was sitting on the low garden wall. His tears had gone, though his eyes were still red.

'My woodwork wasn't much good,' he said, forcing a smile.

'You're just like me, Tommy,' I replied and, putting down my case, I told him all about my egg holder.

*   *   *

Following Mrs Williams' directions, I set off back up the valley. The main road curved gently around a sparsely wooded hill and, where it flattened, a narrow lane, partly hidden by high hedges, led away to the right by an old slate-roofed barn. It was more of a cutting than a lane, for the track was deeply rutted, leaving a high, grassy central ridge along which the little Ford rubbed uneasily. I was afraid my exhaust pipe might come adrift, but was wary of stopping in case, straddled on the prominence, I would fail to get going again.

Steep banks rose at each side, covered with lank brown grass and topped with tangled hedges, shaggy with strands of dead convolvulus. A solitary jay fled out, flashing its white flecked tail as it swooped ahead, as if to warn whoever lived beyond of my intrusion.

It was all a bit unnerving.

The access to the field at the head of the track was guarded by a five-barred gate, green with mould. I had difficulty in unlatching the rusty clasp and, when I did, the gate sagged like a partly collapsed deck chair. It proved awkward and obstinate to open, as if trying to take revenge by straining the muscles of all who wished to pass.

Once inside the field, the going was easier. A dozen sheep had collected around a wooden rack, the top protected by a corrugated sheet to keep the hay dry. There appeared to be three distinct types of sheep: the nervous, the inquisitive and the unconcerned. The nervous looked startled at my presence and scampered away. The inquisitive came cautiously forward a few paces, then stood silently, fixing me with their glassy eyes. While the unconcerned and probably most sensible, concentrated on eating as much as they could while their fellows were distracted.

At the far end there was a gap in the hedgerow where the gate, having succumbed to decay, lay alongside like a crumpled skeleton. Beyond it, the track ran steeply downwards and out of sight. Discretion being the better part of valour, I decided to leave the car and, taking my case and the rope halter, set off in search of Howell Powell and the lame cow.

I hadn't walked far, when a cluster of farm buildings came into view. They were low and stone built, with ancient slit windows, which over the years must have kept both bad weather and uninvited guests firmly at bay. My ears detected the laboured chugging of a tractor and, as I rounded the barn, I discovered it to be an old Fordson, one of the basic mechanical work horses of the war years — sturdy but temperamental.

Crouched over the exposed guts of the vibrating machine, back towards me, and obviously concentrating on some vital adjustment, was my client.

'Hello!' I called. 'Mr Powell!' But my voice made little impact over the chugging engine.

'HELLO!' I repeated, as loudly as I could.

There followed a small explosion and an orange flame, chased eagerly by a cloud of black smoke, shot out from the vertical exhaust pipe. The engine faltered momentarily, so that the tractor ceased juddering, then it seemed to cough and the chassis recovered its frenzied, jerking motion.

Despite the sudden retort, the crouched figure never budged, so I approached until I was directly behind him. I was raising my hand to tap his shoulder when I suddenly realised the import of the situation.

I was now standing behind someone who, living in the depths of the isolated countryside, completely unaware of my presence and certainly not used to visitors, might at the least have an epileptic fit or even a heart attack in response to my touch. I stood for a while, my thoughts practically drowned by the deafening chatter of the engine. Better, I thought, if I withdrew a few feet and waited until he had finished.

I took two steps backward and trod upon a dog.

The poor creature let out such an ear-splitting shriek that it was I who nearly succumbed to apoplexy and all but collapsed in my tracks.

When I had recovered my composure, Howell Powell was standing facing me.

'Sorry,' I apologised weakly. ' I . . . I didn't want to scare you — so I trod on your dog!'

Howell Powell looked somewhat bemused, for by then there was no dog to be seen.

'You all right?' he boomed, his voice sounding louder in the now exaggerated silence.

'Yes,' I replied. 'Just didn't want to frighten you.'

'No,' he said, a trifle vaguely, still not clear as to what had really happened.

'Come to see the lame cow,' I explained, gathering my breath.

He nodded. 'She's in the shed.' And without further ceremony he led off.

'How long has she been lame?' I asked, as I followed him across the yard.

'A week,' he replied, without so much as a turn of his head.

'Tried any treatment yourself?' I enquired.

He opened a stable door and peered inside. 'The sod!' he said.

'What's the matter?' I queried, looking into the stable, not knowing what to expect. As it was, I could see no reason for his blasphemy, for the large cock-horned Ayrshire cow that stood before us seemed quite inoffensive as she unconcernedly picked at some rather coarse hay. Howell Powell studied me quizzically.

'The sod,' he repeated. 'The sod for "foul"!'

It was no good pretending and I told him flatly, I didn't understand.

Had I put a pound in his hand, I could not have changed his attitude so significantly. His gruff manner vanished and he pushed back his tattered cap and smiled.

'You never 'eard of the sod treatment for "foul of the foot"? Well, you ain't no Black Mountain man an' that's for sure.'

I shook my head.

'Fancy that,' he went on. Then his face took on a serious expression, as if it had just registered that I was new. 'You ain't been to me afore, 'ave you?'

'No,' I admitted.

'Where d'you come from?' he enquired, suspiciously.

'I come from Abergranog,' I replied. 'Hugh Lasgarn's the name.'

'You'm a Welshman then,' beamed Howell Powell. 'Well, that's different. You listen, young man, an' I'll tell you all about it.' With that, he folded his arms and stared up at the lintel of the stable door. I realised that it was going to be an explanation in some detail, so I put down the case and halter and leaned against the wall.

'The Black Mountain remedy,' he began, 'has been known in these parts for years. You must watch where the sick beast treads and cut a sod from the very spot it plants the poisoned foot. Then, at night, when the moon is awasting, you throws the sod high in a blackthorn tree.' Howell Powell then shut his eyes, as if about to mutter an incantation.

'As the sod wastes,' he whispered, 'so will the foul disappear.' Then, as if drained of emotion, he stood, eyes closed for quite a while, until I ventured a comment.

'But it didn't work,' I said.

He woke, startled from his reverie.

'Moon was wrong,' he retorted sourly. 'She'll need one of those injections'.

I moved inside the stable to take a closer look at the offending foot. The old cow was certainly lame, for she rested very gingerly on the points of her left hind leg and moved back uneasily when I tried to make her take weight upon it.

'It's not swollen enough for foul,' I remarked, as I carefully ran my hand down the limb and on to the foot where I pressed my finger between the clees.

'Not very tender either, and doesn't smell.' For the foul-producing germ gave rise to a very distinctive obnoxious odour, whence the condition derived its name. 'We'll have to get the foot up.'

Howell Powell puffed and shook his head. 'Bit of a performance, that'll be. She might look sweet and she'll let you touch it, but Bronwen's a cantankerous old witch if she's a mind. You try liftin' 'er foot an' she'll go mad!'

At that, the old cow looked round and all but nodded her spiky head, as if to confirm Howell Powell's comment.

'That new injection works, don' it?' he asked.

'Certainly it does,' I declared, 'but only if the foul is uncomplicated. Penicillin will kill the foul germ, but it's useless if there's a stick, stone or piece of gravel in the foot.'

'Well she won't let you look at it,' Howell asserted emphatically. 'So it's a waste of time you tryin'!'

'Let's put her down,' I suggested.

'What! Not our Bronwen!' he said, incredulously.

'On the floor, rope her so that I can give the foot a thorough examination,' I explained, suddenly realising he thought I intended a more severe solution. 'Have you got a wagon rope?'

'Several.'

'Bring two,' I requested. 'One long and one short.'

Howell Powell fetched the ropes and together we put the halter on his cow and tied her to an iron ring in the wall. I then made a running noose in the long wagon rope and placed it over Bronwen's menacing horns, bringing the trailing end back and winding it around her neck. Then I looped it at the top and took it back behind her shoulders.

'Stand on the other side,' I ordered. 'When I give you the

rope, you pass it back to me under her belly.' In this way, I made two more loops, one behind her forelegs and another in front of the udder, with the trailing end running free behind, so that she looked tied up like a Christmas parcel.

'Now, if we both pull on this free end at the back of her,' I announced, 'the rope will tighten and down she'll go!'

Howell Powell who, so far, had followed every move I had made without a word, eyed me suspiciously. Then he looked at Bronwen, who seemed quite mystified, herself, by the whole performance, shook his head and took hold of the rope.

'When I say "pull".' He nodded. Together we took the strain.

'PULL!'

We heaved in unison and, to my delight, Bronwen first sank to her knees, then her hind quarters wavered and she rolled gently on to one side.

Howell Powell looked at me in amazement.

'Now there's a trick, mun,' he muttered. 'There's a trick.'

'Puts pressure on the spine, just like someone pinching you in the back,' I explained. 'As long as you keep pulling, she can't get up.'

I then took the shorter wagon rope and tied it around the affected limb, pulling it out for examination. While Howell Powell kept the body rope taut, I took my hoof knife and cleaned the foot. As I cleared the heel, Bronwen pulled back sharply and the knife grated against something metallic. I turned the foot slightly to find the head of a rusty nail protruding from the heel. Easing it clear of the flesh with my blade, I took a hold and pulled the nail out with my fingers.

'It wasn't the moon that was wrong,' I called, over my shoulder. 'It was this!' And I held up the nail for him to see.

I cleaned and dressed the wound. 'Now I'll give her an injection. It will stop any infection developing. We don't want Bronwen going wrong again.'

Following treatment, I removed the ropes and the old cow obligingly got to her feet.

Howell Powell carefully examined the offending nail.

'Wasn't fair to the sod treatment, that,' he commented thoughtfully. 'Weren't meant for that.'

'That old remedy is just an excuse,' I chided. 'It's a darn sight easier to sling a lump of mud up into a blackthorn tree than to get the foot up. That's the real sod.'

'No it ain't.' Howell Powell frowned morosely, as he spoke. 'Don' you never make fun of the Mountain, Mr Lasgarn,' he said, in serious tone. ''E's been there a long time.'

I felt slightly put down by his remarks and he must have realised it, for he suddenly clapped his hands and said:

'Well, well. Now I don't suppose you be married.'

'No,' I replied.

'Who looks after you, then?'

'I'm in digs at Putsley.'

'Then you shall 'ave something for your dinner,' he said. 'Jus' you wait 'ere.'

While he was away, I coiled up the ropes and wondered what my reward was going to be. Already I had my Welsh cakes. Some butter would be fine, or eggs, or even a slice of home-cured ham. But my grandiose expectations were shortlived, for Howell Powell soon returned.

''E're, Mr Lasgarn,' he said. 'I be most grateful for what you've done. Take these 'ome with you, they be real tasty.'

And into my hands he put two large, round swedes, which must have weighed all of three pounds each. I couldn't remember if it was one of C. J. Pink's Laws or a piece of McBean's advice, but someone had urged me never to refuse a gift from a farmer, or it would be the last I was offered.

I thanked Howell Powell for the swedes and told him to let me know if Bronwen suffered any setback. Then, I commenced my walk back up the bank.

By the time I reached the car, after humping my medical

140

case, halter and the two swedes, I was exhausted and, throwing my rewards into the passenger well, sat sideways on the seat until I regained my wind.

A glance at my watch showed it was past two o'clock, and I realised I should be on my way.

The green mould gate was equally truculent on the outward journey, and when I eventually dragged it back into place, one of the bars came adrift; as I picked it up I spied two nails, similar to the one in Bronwen's foot. So much for Howell Powell's folk medicine.

'Never make fun of the Mountain!' I shouted at the top of my voice, mimicking in exaggerated Welsh, Howell Powell's terse advice.

As the car lurched down the lane, the swedes rolled about hysterically beside me. Keeping my right hand on the wheel, I bent over to put them on the seat where they would be more stable, but my bodily movement jerked the steering and the wheels jarred on the central ridge of the track. The little Ford bucked like a mustang and, in attempting control, I over-corrected, causing it to leap out of the ruts and drift onto its left side.

It was still going forward at a perilous angle until, with a bang and a shudder, the little car came to rest with both offside wheels in the ditch. With some difficulty, I scrambled out and, hands on hips, surveyed my predicament. Well and truly wedged; there was no way I was going to extricate my vehicle without help.

I trudged back up the track and for the third time dragged open the green mould gate. As I did, I glanced upwards at the Black Mountain.

The mist had risen, clearing the summit and leaving a narrow orange gap of hazy sunlight between it and the overhanging cloud. It looked just like a grinning mouth.

'All right, we're quits now,' I shouted irritably, and set off across the field to enlist the aid of Howell Powell and his fiery Fordson.

Howell Powell showed little surprise at my return, as if he was half expecting it. At a frustratingly slow pace, he collected the short wagon rope, started up the tractor and came back with me.

'Wonder what frightened 'er?' he commented sarcastically as he surveyed my up-ended car. 'You'll 'ave to cut 'er oats down, Mr Lasgarn, that's what you'll 'ave to do.'

*   *   *

It was nearly two hours later that I arrived at 'Top Shop' at St Madoc's. It was right by the roadside, with a small iron fence across its front.

'Evan P. Evans General Stores,' announced the wording above the door. A blackhandled 'sit up and beg' bicycle leaned against the railings — a lady's model with a string guard over the rear wheel. Behind it, fixed to the gate, was a sign that stated quite emphatically and with typical Welsh double emphasis, 'No Parking By Here'.

'Top Shop' was part of a double-fronted cottage which, from its entrance, led into a narrow passage barred halfway by a low gate, on which was another sign, reading 'Private'.

On the right was a door; two signs here: 'Shop' and 'No Dogs'.

I opened the door and entered, to find myself in a room jam-packed to the ceiling with goods. The free floor space was already occupied by two people: A woman in a black coat and shiny black straw hat, who was counting out coins from her purse onto the counter, and a wizened little man, in a cap, tattered rain coat and oversized wellington boots. His face was red as a cherry, with a film of white, whiskery hairs covering his cheeks.

There were open sacks of sugar and flour and hams hanging down, a great bacon slicer with a shining circular knife, cheeses of all varieties and a mountain of butter on a marble slab. Palethorpe's sausages, brawn and cooked meats fought for display behind, whilst above, the shelves were packed to capacity with teas, coffees, syrups and jams. There were cakes on a tiered cake stand, jars of sweets and Lovell's King Rex Toffees. At my back stood a glass-fronted cupboard containing health cures, salts, lineaments and pills. There was hardware, software, footwear and well, you name it, it was all there — somewhere — and the mix of aromas, scents and smells defied description.

Standing beaming benevolently across the counter, white-aproned, black-waistcoated, with black tie and little cutty-back collar, was the proprietor of the multi-purpose rural emporium, Evan P. Evans.

My entrance caused an immediate tension in the atmosphere. The woman with the coins eyed me suspiciously over the rims of her spectacles and the old gent attempted to tuck himself in between two sugar bags, while Evan P. Evans rubbed his hands together eagerly, in the manner of all shopkeepers, and continued smiling. At that point, one of the woman's coins rolled from the counter onto the floor and the three of us bent down to retrieve it; being in such tight compass, we all but collided and stood up without anyone picking it up. I bent down again to collect it, replacing it with the rest. The joint action seemed to break the ice and suddenly everyone became good companions.

'Don't throw it away, Mrs Baggot,' said the old gent.

'No fear of that, Mr Preece,' she replied. 'Too 'ard to come by.' And turning to me she said, 'Thank you,' then stood back, motioning me to squeeze up to the counter.

'I'd like to use the 'phone, please,' I explained. 'I'm a vet. Mr McBean from Hacker's said it would be all right.'

'Most certainly you can, Mr . . .'

'Lasgarn. Hugh Lasgarn.'

'Sorry to hear about Mr Hacker's death.' Evan P. Evans lowered his voice. 'He was a fine man,' he said, reverently. 'A fine man.'

'Saved a mare for me last year. Remember that grey mare, Evan?' the old gent interjected. 'Came in the middle of the night to 'er.'

'Yes,' I said. 'He'll be missed very much indeed.'

No one spoke further and they all stood, heads bowed,

143

for about a minute. It was most touching and I think they would have stood much longer had I not shuffled and cleared my throat.

'The telephone?' I enquired, quietly.

'Through here,' said Evan, still in slightly funereal tone, and drew back a curtain that had hidden the access to an adjoining room. 'Who would you like to call?' he asked, smiling inquisitively.

'The surgery.'

'Oh, yes. 'O' for operator, then give your number.'

The telephone, which stood in pride of place on a mahogany stand, was covered with a sort of woollen tea cosy on which was embroidered in rainbow colours the word 'TELEPHONE'.

I got through to the operator and, whilst she was connecting me, I realised the conversation in the adjoining shop had ceased. Remembering McBean's advice and the wartime slogan 'Walls have ears', I decided to be careful in what I said.

McBean came through and I explained why I had been held up.

'As long as you are all right, Hugh, that's the main thing,' he replied. 'Just one call for you on the way back. Hinks of Greenmore. Cow calved last week and not cleansed the afterbirth. It'll be a bit of a stinker I'm afraid, we normally like them at twenty-four hours, but old Hinks always hopes they'll drop away by themselves and save a visit.' He gave me directions to Greenmore. 'There's nothing else, so you might as well go back to your digs and have a bath — you'll no doubt need one after that job. I'll see to the small animals, you can have tonight off.'

The call finished, I paid Evan P. Evans the shilling he requested.

Mrs Baggot had gone, but old Mr Preece was still there.

'Know anything about dogs?' he questioned.

'A little,' I declared.

'Why does my old sheepdog shake 'er 'ead?'

'Bad ears,' I suggested.

144

'Could be,' he said, nodding. 'What can I do for that?'

'Olive oil,' I replied.

'Olive oil!'

'Yes, up there, next to the mustard,' I pointed to the third shelf. 'Warm it up, a few drops down the ear, do the trick.'

And with that slick piece of diagnosis and advice, I bid them both 'Good Day'.

But, my 'devil may care' progress was sharply arrested when I got outside, for lying beneath the front of my car was a large pool of rusty water — the radiator had leaked. I had known that it was faulty, but regular daily topping had so far been sufficient. I checked the hoses, but they were sound, and concluded that the episode in Howell Powell's ditch had aggravated the condition; so back into 'Top Shop' I went, to explain my predicament.

Evan was very sympathetic and went away to get some water.

'Know anything about radiators?' I jovially asked Mr Preece.

'A little,' he said, rubbing his teeth with the stem of a well-smoked briar pipe.

'What can I do for it?' I asked.

'Mustard,' he replied.

'Mustard!'

'Ay. Up there, next to the olive oil,' he grinned. 'Put it in your radiator, mix it up, do the trick.'

'You're pulling my leg,' I said incredulously.

'No, 'e's right,' said Evan, who had returned with a watering can. 'Mix it in with the water, it'll stop the leak. Get you back to Ledingford, anyway.'

Sure enough, two tins of Coleman's down the spout under Mr Preece's direction, and I was on my way. One good turn deserves another I thought, and I hoped that Mr Preece's sheepdog would respond as well as my little Ford.

McBean, I thought, had been very decent in giving me the night off and I welcomed the offer. But it was when my eye rested upon the two large round swedes, bobbing up and down gently on the seat alongside me, that I suddenly remembered Miss Lafont.

It was Friday — she was going tonight. If I got cracking I could be back in time. But, following my encounter with Hinks' cow, my aroma would be far from conducive to laying on the charm. Dammit!

McBean was a clever devil! Have the night off, indeed!

As I drove back towards Ledingford, I glimpsed the Black Mountain receding in my mirror. The cloud had risen and the evening sun glowed softly above its purple summit — it really was a beautiful sight and I resolved there and then, for several reasons, 'not to make fun of the Mountain' again.

*   *   *

I concluded my second week with a very busy Saturday and was thankful when evening came. Not that the day was without its satisfaction, for I had my radiator fixed at the garage, successfully delivered two sets of twin lambs, reduced a blown cow with my probang and visited Mrs Williams at Pontavon, where, although one more calf had died, the others seemed likely to survive. Finally, I had called at five farms on the 'Mastitis Run'.

The 'Mastitis Run', or 'Tit Trot' as McBean rudely termed it, was a series of farm visits at evening milking for the purpose of treating infected udders. Penicillin and streptomycin were available in crystalline form and, diluted in sterile water, were injected up the teat canal of the ailing quarter on three evening milkings. Successive visits were necessary due to the instability of the diluted antibiotic and the fact that the drug was not freely available to the farmers. It was, indeed, a 'whistle-stop' tour of the dairy herds, often seeing only the backside of the cowman as he carried on with his milking.

It was simple: stop car, into cowshed, make up solution,

squirt up teat, back into car and off.

I returned to my digs just before seven o'clock. Charlie was out and Brad had waited to rustle up ham and eggs for me, before going off to visit her old folk. After my supper I carried the dishes through to the tiny kitchen, rinsed them and stacked them on the draining board, then I settled down in the deep armchair by the fire in the lounge.

On the opposite chair, in a most unusual posture, lay Percy, the larger of Brad's two cats. What a lesson in relaxation was provided by a cat, I mused. Sleek, speedy and agile when hunting, custom-built for the job, but when off duty their bodies became loose and pliable, melting luxuriously into the contour of any resting place they cared to choose. Percy's rear half lay in the centre of the seat, upside down, with his legs pointing upwards, but sagging. The middle of his body, however, had swivelled so that his chest was upright with right foreleg tucked beneath and, to complete the contortion, his head and left leg hung lifelessly down towards the floor.

Yet, despite this seemingly impossible position, his eyes were tightly closed and he purred deeply and with immense satisfaction.

I lay back in my seat and in a much simpler way, tried to emulate him.

Percy's example had the required soporific effect, for it was over one hour and a half later that I awoke to the scratching of a key in the front door lock. It was Brad returning from visiting, and already Percy had left his chair to greet her. She popped her woolly-hatted head around the door and chastised me gently for letting the fire sink so low. Then, she retired to the kitchen, to re-appear shortly with a cup of cocoa, served as always, very correctly, on a blue tray with matching napkin.

Warmed and contented, I decided to turn in. The sideboard clock chimed eleven and, as it ended, the telephone rang.

It was Miss Billings, her voice soft and apologetic — how

she had altered since first we met. She was now in residence with the late Mr Hacker's widow and took all the telephone messages at night.

'I'm sorry, Mr Lasgarn, but it's a calving at Mr Ridway of Beckley. Apparently she's been trying since milking time, but without success. Do you know Beckley?'

'Yes,' I replied. 'I passed through there on Tuesday.'

'Well,' she explained, 'Mr Ridway farms at The Beeches. Go past the church and follow the lane to the end.'

The call noted, I decided a good wash was required to freshen up and popped up to the bathroom.

When I came down again, Brad added her commiserations at my misfortune in being called out.

'You wrap up warm, now,' she advised in a motherly way. 'Bitter out, it is.'

Taking her advice, I was donning my duffle and scarf when the door opened and in walked Charlie.

A Jack-in-the-box could not have presented a more startling entry, for my Cockney companion was attired in a loud mustard-yellow suit, the jacket of which sported highly exaggerated shoulders and a wide black velvet collar. The trouser legs were like drain-pipes and terminated a good eight inches above black, thick-soled, suede shoes. The gap between exposed bright green socks, so dazzling as to cause instant disturbance of vision when they met the eye. His hair, heavily greased, was slicked back in the Elvis style and his cheeks appeared unusually red.

'Wotcher, Hubert!' he shouted jovially, slapping me on the shoulder with one hand and shutting the door behind him with the other. An aroma of heavy aftershave and whisky filled the hallway. Charlie stood rather unsteadily before me, casting his eyes over my scarf and duffle coat, down to my boots and back up again. 'On the night shift, Hubert?' he enquired. I nodded. 'Where you goin' then?' he asked blearily.

'Cow calving at Beckley,' I replied.

'Like some company?' he asked, brushing back his hair

with both hands.

'What, you?' I responded, with some amazement.

Charlie's hands slowly dropped from his head, slid around his face and finished up clasped in front of his chest. 'Well, I wasn't thinking of fixin' you up with a bird, Hubert,' he said, looking quite forlorn.

'Oh. You can come, if you like,' I rejoined. 'But you'd better change first.'

'Change!' exclaimed Charlie. 'Ain't this gear Country Style?'

'Not exactly,' I admitted.

'Well, I'm only goin' to watch, ain't I?' he said, his face beaming with delight. 'Come on, Hubert. Let's get cracking!'

With my somewhat inebriated passenger just about aboard, I set off for Beckley. The first turning from the digs was sharp and right-handed and as I swung the little Ford, the passenger seat, which was loose, slipped sideways, nearly depositing Charlie in my lap.

'Blimey, Hubert!' he gasped, recovering himself. 'Proper little dolly-trap you've got here, my son. You're a dark horse, Hubert, an' no mistake.' He then proceeded to fumble in his pockets, grunting and puffing as he did so. 'Mind if I smoke?' he asked, after he had managed to find his cigarettes and lighter.

'Not at all,' I said.

With some difficulty, he lit up. 'Went out on the town, tonight,' he explained. 'Finished up at the Three Ravens Club. Met a friend of yours there an' all.'

'A friend of mine?' I questioned, wondering who on earth it could be.

'Very smart little piece. Thinks you're "wonderfool"!' he threw back his head and chuckled. 'Got a little pooch called Petal.'

'Miss Lafont,' I said.

'Call me Mimi!' said Charlie, in a mock French accent. 'Disappointed you didn't give her the treatment last night.

149

Some Mick saw her.'

'McBean,' I replied. 'Yes, she had an appointment, but I had other calls.'

'Said I'd take you down there one night,' he continued. 'Have a bit of a knees up. You get the night off — do you good.'

'Look forward to it,' I said, but as we rattled on our way to Beckley, I pondered his suggestion with mixed feelings.

The village was deserted as we drove through. Bearing right at the green to the church, we followed the lane to the end where a gate across the road bore a sign: 'The Beeches'.

'I'll do it,' offered Charlie, and was out of the car before I could even remind him to watch his step. After some fiddling, he unlatched the gate and heaved it open, then, turning to face the lights, swept his right arm downwards and stamped his feet in a grand matadorial gesture, before beckoning me through.

I sighed unconsciously. Help at night calving cases was always acceptable, but I wondered what reception I would get from the Ridways with a half-cut Cockney in a mustard-yellow suit and black suede shoes.

Charlie closed the gate and caught up. As soon as he climbed in, I sensed the pungent odour of cow dung and realised that my helpmate had already garnished himself with something distasteful — but as he made no comment, neither did I.

The track across the fields was fairly smooth and Charlie opened two more gates before we arrived at a cluster of buildings sitting on the highest point of the farm, like a small fort. The farmhouse door was open and, as we drew near, I saw, silhouetted in the opening, the figure of a very large lady.

'Phew!' exclaimed Charlie, catching sight of her. 'You won't get many of those to the pound, Hubert. Ain't she a whopper!'

Indeed she was, and as we were parked on an upward

slope, it accentuated her perspective considerably. What a contrast to Mimi Lafont, for Mrs Ridway, if it were she, was straight from the 'Ride of the Valkyries', a Wagnerian soprano if ever I saw one; had she burst into song it would have seemed most natural.

'You stay here,' I said to Charlie, hopefully.

'I'll come with you, Hubert,' he replied in a hoarse whisper. 'Just in case.'

Clambering out of the car, I approached the warrior maiden. She was not unattractive, just large in every department. Long dark hair flowed down over the shoulders of her rough, smock-type dress which was quite flattering to her contours; but so massive were her breasts that, as she gazed down upon me, it was as if she was looking over a precipice.

'Mrs Ridway?' I enquired. She nodded, but her features remained expressionless. 'The vet. Hugh Lasgarn.'

Suddenly, without warning, like a giant hippo, she moved. Her eyes widened fearfully and she raised her hands, clasped them to her formidable chest and gave a high-pitched shriek. I froze on the spot.

Then I realised that Charlie had arrived out of the darkness alongside me.

'This is Mr Love. A friend of mine — from London,' I added, trying to make the introduction sound more descriptive than excusing.

'Evenin' darlin',' called Charlie in his casual way. 'Nice night for a ride in the country. Where's the action, then?'

Mrs Ridway stood before us, nervously massaging her ample thighs and breathing heavily. 'My man's with the cow,' she said, in a surprisingly high-pitched tone. 'Over there in the boosie.'

'The where?' said Charlie, chuckling to himself.

'Cowhouse!' I retorted under my breath. 'It's country slang.'

Mrs Ridway pointed to a building next to the house from where the glow of a lamp was flickering through the narrow windows.

'Right,' said Charlie, clapping his hands. 'You get the kettle on, darlin', we'll pop to the boosie and get the job done. What do we want, Hubert?'

'You're sure you wouldn't prefer to stay in the car?' I suggested to him quietly, for his exuberance was beginning to worry me.

'Not a bit of it, my old son,' he replied, slapping me across the back. 'What can I carry?'

Back at the car, I gave him the metal calving box, put on my wellington boots, stripped off my shirt and drew on my 'mucklets', and together we entered the dimly lit building.

Mr Ridway was small in stature compared with his wife, but his amazement when confronted with Charlie and myself considerably exceeded hers. For a moment, when we appeared, I thought he was going to climb up the wall.

'My God!' he gasped, practically putting his hands in the air. 'W-who are you?'

Men from Mars could not have created a more dramatic entry. However, after I made the introductions, he calmed down, but kept giving sideways glances at Charlie, who by now had rolled up his trouser legs in anticipation of the 'action'.

The cow was a Guernsey type, not very large and jigging about uneasily in her stall. A dark shadow fell upon us as Mrs Ridway arrived, surprisingly silently, carrying a bucket of hot water, soap and towel. So it was, with Mr Ridway holding the tail and his wife and Charlie in close attendance, that I commenced my examination.

Carefully I probed the soft vaginal passage, through the dilated cervix, over the pelvic brim and into the womb. 'See with your fingers,' C. J. Pink had said, and how true that was proving to be. The membranes had burst some time previously, although the area was still well lubricated, but as I searched and 'saw' I could appreciate no head or legs; instead my hand rested upon a bony prominence from the tip of which sprouted an unmistakable structure — a tail.

I withdrew my arm and straightened my back; the eyes of my silent audience studied me intently.

'Coming backwards,' I announced. 'Breech presentation.'

'Awkward, Hubert?' asked Charlie solemnly.

'The back legs are forward,' I explained, 'making the presented end larger than normal. Rather like trying to push a cork into a bottle.'

'You'll have to turn it, then?' he asked.

'Not enough room for that, even though the calf is not very large. No, I shall have to try and bring the hind legs back up.'

Soaping my arms thoroughly, I re-introduced them into the vagina and, standing behind the extremely patient mother, passed my hands forward onto the unborn calf's rump. Pushing onwards with my left hand, I delved inwards and downwards over its hip, alongside the bent hock, until my fingers just clasped the points of the toes of the left foot. Once I had grasped it, I took a deep breath and rested for a moment.

'You all right?' asked Charlie urgently.

'Thanks,' I replied. 'I've got one foot, next job is to get it up.'

That was the most delicate part of the operation, turning the leg to bring it into a posterior position. The wall of the womb was of unbelievable texture when one considered its elasticity and strength, and its resistance to gradual, even pressure was considerable. But sharp jabs, such as could readily be made by the point of a hock or the rim of a hoof, could rip the womb like a knife through butter. I knew that, as I drew the foot backwards, the hock would automatically rise, and if my movement was too rough or the cow strained at the wrong moment, I could rupture the wall immediately.

'Pinch her back,' I ordered. 'It stops the straining.'

Mrs Ridway stepped forward and dropped her large hands across the Guernsey's spine.

Gently I pulled on the foot and bent the hock, keeping

153

the points of the toes deep in the palm of my hand. Pushing the buttocks forward with my other hand to create as much free space as possible, I drew the leg slowly backwards — and upwards — and sideways — and straight.

With a sigh of relief, I brought the foot into view.

'Well done, Hubert!' shouted Charlie excitedly, his suedes squelching in the wet straw. 'Get the other, my son!'

After some more gentle persuasion, I did get the other one and then roped both legs securely, attaching the wooden handles.

By now, Charlie had discarded his yellow jacket and rolled up both sleeves ready to pull. It was indeed an odd scene, with the great Mrs Ridway on one rope and Cockney Charlie on the other, for Mr Ridway still clung firmly to the Guernsey's tail.

'When I say "pull",' I ordered, and Charlie and Mrs Ridway took the strain. Even then, he couldn't resist a quip, for he gently nudged the well-endowed lady in the ribs and called out: 'What's a nice girl like you doin' in a dirty old shed like this?' At which Mrs Ridway's seemingly expressionless face broke into a smile and she burst into laughter.

The delivery was smooth, and a perfect bull calf soon lay glistening in the straw. I slapped its chest and it drew its legs up short. I slapped it again and it repeated the action.

'What's wrong with him?' asked Charlie.

'He's not breathing,' I replied sharply. 'Pick him up by his back legs and shake him.' Hurriedly, I took one leg and Charlie the other, and we jerked the little chap up and down. 'Fluid on his chest. Backwards calves often suffer from this,' I explained.

Three times we tried, but he wouldn't breathe.

'Try some straw,' suggested Mr Ridway and, taking a piece from the bedding on the floor, tickled the calf's nostrils, but there was no response.

I got down on my knees and, placing one hand over the

calf's nose, blew down into its mouth in an attempt to stimulate respiration.

It was useless and I felt about the same. I could hear the heart eagerly thumping in the little bull's chest, but I knew that if the lungs failed, it would soon cease to function. Despairingly I looked up at Charlie; his face was quite white, the ruddiness of his earlier complexion vanished. Suddenly, his face lit up and he clenched his fists, shook them vigorously in the air and shouted: 'COLD WATER! WHERE'S SOME COLD WATER?'

'There's a trough outside,' shouted back Mr Ridway, getting the second shock of the night at Charlie's outburst.

'Pick him up, Hubert,' roared Charlie, grabbing the calf's forelegs.

I was quite taken aback by his action and for a moment stood motionless.

'Pick him up,' he shouted at me again. 'An' open the door, darlin!' he called to Mrs Ridway.

We swung the calf outside and up to the trough. 'IN!' bellowed Charlie. 'ALL OF HIM!' And with that, we plunged the newborn calf deep into the icy water.

The little bull gasped audibly as we pulled him out and hauled him back to the shed. As he lay in the straw I could see his chest heaving and I set to, rubbing him with a wisp until he was breathing deeply and evenly. Soon he was shaking his head and finally bawled out lustily, so that I ceased my rubbing and sat back on my haunches with relief.

'I never seen that afore,' exclaimed Mr Ridway, shaking Charlie by the hand. 'Where did you ever learn a trick like that?'

'Saw John Wayne do it on a ranch in Nevada,' said Charlie. 'Couple of years ago.'

'Well, I never,' commented Mr Ridway. 'Fancy that.'

I looked hard at Charlie, but he had already turned his attentions to Mrs Ridway. 'I couldn't 'arf go a nice cuppa, darlin,' he was saying, and Mrs Ridway, now all smiles and chuckles, said: 'Certainly you shall, Mr Charlie.

Certainly.' And with that, she bustled off to the house.

'Come on, Hubert,' he called over his shoulder, giving me a broad wink as he did so. 'Let's get this show on the road.'

We sat in the kitchen drinking tea laced generously with whisky, and eating thick ham sandwiches which Mrs Ridway soon prepared. Charlie was on top form, cracking jokes and singing Cockney rhymes with the Ridways joining in lustily — it really was quite a party.

It was well into the small hours when we left, bearing a dozen eggs each, a thick wedge of home-cured bacon and a pint of cream.

When we got to the last gate on the edge of the farm, Charlie closed it wearily and clambered back into the car.

'Smudged the old finery a bit,' he said, surveying the sleeves of his jacket in the dashboard light.

'Sorry about that, Charlie,' I apologised. 'But you really did save that calf tonight. Thanks.'

'Think nothing of it, my old son,' he replied, generously.

'But why did you tell them you saw John Wayne do it in Nevada?' I asked. 'You've never been to the States.'

'Course, I haven't,' he chortled. 'Course, I haven't, but I've been to the Odeon in Leicester Square, ain't I?' With that, he slapped me hard over the shoulders. 'Drive on, Hubert,' he shouted. 'Drive on!'

Six

During my early days in country practice, I found the transition from student to veterinary surgeon, although abrupt, not as obvious as I might have expected. This factor was due in some measure to the change in circumstances occasioned by Mr Hacker Senior's unfortunate demise and the pressure of work that consequently ensued. Such that I had little time to be truly aware of what was happening. But even despite this unfortunate turn of fate, there would have been more than enough to occupy my mind in the absolute diversity of the lifestyle.

Newborn lawyers, doctors, teachers and engineers commence their careers in regulated circumstances and within predictable surroundings of offices, wards, classrooms or building sites. But for a young vet in country practice, places of work can range from windswept hills and river pastures to dark, animal-warm cowsheds, stately homes or even gypsy encampments; and there are demands, not only upon academic knowledge, but upon physical stamina, ingenuity, diplomacy and above all, one's sense of humour.

In my first three weeks, I dealt with what seemed like a multitude of species and breeds of varying size, colour and condition, and, as well as my patients, I also encountered a glorious mix of humanity, as varied as the stock I treated. There was, however, one marked difference between the animals and those who owned or cared for them, for while the former's colour, shape and breeding capacity were far more diverse than my own species, they could not talk. I soon realised this obvious difference put vets in a very special position when it came to communication.

'Talk, touch and treat them as equal,' C. J. Pink had said, and how right he was; except that with practically every animal I saw, there was a human spokesman or spokeswoman, and it was often this third party who presented the greatest problem.

Take Miss Millicent for example.

She was a tall, angular, spinster lady, who came to the surgery one evening carrying a friendly little tortoiseshell cat, called Sybil.

'She doesn't seem to be quite herself,' commented Miss Millicent, placing Sybil upon the examination table. 'She seems rather dreamy.'

Now, 'dreamy' was not a clinical description of a symptom, but I understood what she meant.

'She eats extremely well, in fact better than she has ever done, and she does everything else quite properly. But lately she doesn't seem so active and sleeps a lot.'

The little cat purred contentedly as I passed my stethoscope over her soft coat. Ears, eyes, mouth were perfect. There were no joint swellings or pain in any part of her body and her temperature was normal. Miss Millicent was right, she was just 'dreamy'.

I gently palpated her abdomen and she whisked her tail, as if disapproving of my familiarity. Then my fingers probed a little deeper and I found the answer. 'She's pregnant,' I announced confidently.

'Impossible,' replied Miss Millicent, equally confidently.

There was a moment when the conversation could have developed into a 'she is', 'she isn't' ding-dong pantomime situation, but I avoided this by lowering my tone and adjusting the stethoscope around my neck to assert my professional authority.

'She is, Miss Millicent. Definitely,' I assured. 'I can feel her distended womb. It's quite distinct. There are at least three and possibly more.'

Miss Millicent looked more puzzled than shocked.

'But she's never been out,' she wailed.

'Perhaps she slipped through an open window,' I suggested.

'I am very careful about windows; wire netting guards each one. The house is very secure. It has to be when you live alone.'

'A door open,' I volunteered.

'I am very careful about doors,' she replied adamantly. 'And the porch is double locked.'

The subject of the investigation curled herself up unconcernedly.

'Impossible,' continued Miss Millicent. 'Impossible.'

I studied the snoozing bundle on the table. 'Any other cats in the house?' I enquired, a trifle vaguely.

Miss Millicent leaned forward and picked up Sybil, cuddling the little tortoiseshell to her flat bosom. 'Only George,' she replied, rubbing her cheek across the soft fur. 'But he's her brother — and he wouldn't do a thing like that!'

Certainly, I was beginning to find that, when speaking on behalf of their pets, owners tended to humanise their companions regarding symptoms, feelings and, in Miss Millicent's case, even morals.

But there were occasions when a case history was presented in more realistic terms and still gave rise to pitfalls, as I discovered when I went to Joe Price's farm at Hill Morton, to carry out a Tuberculin Test.

In the fifties, the Tuberculosis Eradication Scheme was in full swing, in an attempt to eliminate the insidious disease that was rife in both cattle and human populations.

'A disease of great antiquity,' I remembered Professor Bardsley booming during lectures at Glasgow. 'Found in the mummies of Ancient Egypt, it is a disease of community life, disseminated from the centres of ancient culture around the Mediterranean, hence to Europe, the New World — and you!'

Bovine Tuberculosis at the time affected about one third

of all cattle in varying degrees. As well as causing an incurable wasting condition in livestock, it was transmissible to humans through unpasteurised milk and, for the latter reason alone, its eradication was of paramount importance.

The diagnosis and elimination of infected cattle was carried out by means of the single, comparative intradermal sensitivity test, otherwise known as the 'lump test'. This entailed injecting a minute dose of an extract of tuberculosis germs into the neck skin of the animal. The tuberculin, as it was termed, would not cause disease, but stimulated a local reaction which showed up as a swelling. In three days the swelling was measured with calipers, and if it exceeded certain limits, the animal was classed as a reactor and slaughtered.

Two types of tuberculosis extract were used, one derived from poultry germs, called avian, and the other from human germs, called mammalian. The avian was not of serious consequence, being used as a control and given about two inches above the mammalian injection. If the top lump was therefore larger than the bottom, the cow was cleared. So a large top lump was vital to passing the test, and so important that there was often some jiggery-pokery to ensure that it came up to size. Because of its avian origin, there were tales of eggs being fed by the bucketful to cows before testing, and even rumours of more unsavoury poultry derivatives being added to the food, in the hope of ensuring a good top lump.

McBean had told me of one test he carried out, where the condition of the cows pointed very much to a generalised infection with tuberculosis. But the first test showed them to be all clear, for at the reading the top lumps on every cow were very much larger than the bottom ones.

'I thought there was something queer,' McBean explained, 'For the skin was greasy and I could whiff paraffin in the air.' Two clear tests were necessary at an interval of one month, before the herd could be accepted by the Ministry, and on the second test, without informing the farmer, McBean reversed the injections. This would make no difference to the result, other than that the bottom lump was now the control and the top, the failing reaction. At the reading three days later, the top lumps were again the larger and the smell of paraffin still in the air.

'When I told him they had all failed, it was then that he came clean, so he did,' explained McBean. 'The old varmint was injecting paraffin over the area where I had done my test, to make sure it would swell and I would pass them. Not all the crooks are inside prison.'

But Joe Price was of a different mould and as honest as they came. The road to his farm was ancient and well worn and the little Ford's hard-sprung chassis took a severe buffeting.

Joe was waiting on the yard to greet me. A stocky figure, hands deep in the pockets of his patched, brown stock coat. I introduced myself and commented on the change in the weather.

''Tis cold enough for a walking stick,' he said, roaring with laughter at his quip. 'Don't doubt you'll need a hand with the clerking,' he continued. 'Our Ann can see to that.'

Indeed, it was a great help to have someone to record the identification numbers tattooed in the cow's ears and take down the skin measurements, before I gave the injection. And to cap it all, Joe's daughter was really something special; not that she said a lot, but who cared when she had blonde hair, blue eyes and a figure that did all the talking.

The testing went extremely well and by 11.30 we were finished.

'Go along to the house and make a cup of tea for the vet an' me, m'dear,' said Joe to his daughter as I cleared up my tack. 'Us'll be in, shortly.'

I watched her wiggle across the yard and into the kitchen, and as the door closed, old Joe lowered his voice and, in a confidential tone, said:

'Vet, I'd be most obliged if you'd 'ave a look at Ann's

arse afore you go.'

I stood rooted to the ground as medical ethics, in confusion, raced through my mind. In my wildest dreams, I had never expected anything like that, even though I was very deep in the countryside. And as I followed him to the house I wondered, 'Should I?' 'Could I?' 'What would the Min. of Ag. say?'

As we reached the kitchen door, I felt my palms becoming slightly moist, but instead of halting, Joe carried on and turned down a narrow path at the side of the house. There, confronting us, was a stable and, with its head hanging over the door, stood a chestnut hunter with a white blaze.

'Ann's arse,' announced Joe. 'I think 'e's sprained a fetlock!'

So much for human involvement in animal matters, such things that degree courses at university in veterinary medicine and surgery don't cover. Indeed, there are occasions when all the learning is plainly inadequate and the demands not purely academic, but bordering upon the emotional. 'There is no substitute for experience.' Who said it? It could have been Pink, Bardsley or McBean — certainly it was someone who found out the hard way.

Experience is a wisdom derived from the changes and trials of life, an event or course of events by which one is affected. But when the Reverend Gladstone asked for his dog to be put to sleep, for me it was more than just an experience; what it was, I am still not too clear.

Saint Mary's Church, Brentdor, was a building of red and grey sandstone standing upon rising ground, just outside the village. Obscured by tall elm and sycamore, it was not readily visible unless one took the winding lane that led to it and, apart from the vicarage, nowhere else. The vicarage itself, a tall plain dwelling in similar stone with a slate roof and long, narrow windows, lay beyond and was even more obscured by a high hedge of fir trees. The lane terminated in a small turning area, devoid of tarmac and muddy from the previous night's rain.

That morning, I left the car, unlatched the sinking wooden gate and took the path that trailed through an unkempt shrubbery, the foliage hanging heavily in the cold, damp air. The path gave way to a clearing that had once been a lawn, but now resembled a lumpy cow pasture, with clumps of couch grass and dead thistles. The straggling weeds spread beyond the confines of the rough sward, invading flower beds that must have known more orderly growth in bygone days.

As I made for the front door, I felt engulfed in an air of desolation and sadness.

The bell pull responded jerkily and, after an interval during which I imagined wires and rusty wheels wearily transmitting my call, a bell rang faintly within the depths of the house. I waited, clutching my case in a silence broken only by the heavy drips falling irregularly from the sodden leaves. I was on the point of giving the round black knob a second tug, when I was aware of a shuffling sound and, with the drawing of the bolt, the door juddered open.

White hair was the only distinguishing feature, the rest of the frail figure in shabby clerical black and faded collar being hard to distinguish against the drab background, but there was no doubt it was the Reverend Gladstone.

'You've come to see Tess,' he said, quietly. A gentle but sad smile played upon his drawn features and he shivered slightly. 'Come along in,' he beckoned. 'She's in the study.'

I followed the aged cleric across the gloomy hallway. Dark oil paintings in heavy gilt frames hung from the walls and, as I passed a stand laden with an untidy mix of coats and a collection of walking sticks, I noticed some lady's hats hanging at the side. The Reverend Gladstone, sensing my observation, said without turning: 'My dear wife passed away last year, after much suffering. Sadly missed,' he added, shaking his head. 'Sadly missed.'

Turning, he entered the study, a small room with a distinctly musty odour, which I suspected came from a sagging red curtain partly covering the door. More red curtains hung limply on either side of a box window, in the small bay of which stood a rexine sofa, piled high with yellowing newspapers. A glass-doored bookcase with cracked panes, an armchair and two stools stood formally against the other walls, while the centre of the room was occupied by a large mahogany desk littered with books, papers, pens and inks, sweet tins and a collection of bric-a-brac that appeared to have lain undisturbed for some considerable time.

There was only one picture on the wall, fixed over the empty fireplace. It was quite narrow and showed Jesus holding a lantern, emerging from what appeared to be a shrubbery, not unlike the one outside. Beneath it were the words: 'Behold, I am the Light of the World'.

The Reverend Gladstone shuffled his carpet-slippered feet towards the desk and leaned heavily upon it. He appeared to have difficulty in getting his breath and, when he did, he gave a slight cough and then pointed to the floor behind him. There, lying prostrate before a one-bar electric fire, greying muzzle resting upon a green pillow, her body partly covered by a patchwork blanket, was an aged Red Setter.

'Tess,' said the old man affectionately. 'My Tess.'

Putting my case on the floor, I knelt beside the old dog and gently drew back the blanket. Though her coat still shone, she was painfully thin and her flanks slack and hollow. Laying my hand upon her chest I felt her heart thumping irregularly and her breathing, though not distressed, was very shallow.

'She started to falter two days ago,' he began. 'Until then she was eating quite well. Smaller meals than she used to, of course, and she took things a lot slower. Like we all must do,' he sighed. 'For some time she's been drinking more water than usual and I got some tablets for her kidneys. But she is fifteen and I became resigned that nothing could be done.'

Tess lay perfectly still and relaxed, quite oblivious to the discussion, but to me, it was obvious that her resistance was failing fast.

'I'm afraid that, for Tess, things are wearing out. Nothing lasts for ever,' I said.

'How right you are, young man,' replied the Reverend Gladstone. 'How right you are.' He moved unsteadily over to the armchair and, supporting himself upon its side, sat down. 'Fifteen years,' he continued, and his face took on another smile, but this time there was a more obvious thread of happiness in it, as memories of Tess and her companionship came flooding back.

He told me how, with his wife, he had returned from missionary work abroad to take the living at Brentdor.

'We bought her as a pup, when we moved in. She was so full of fun, my wife would play with her for hours on the lawn.' He raised his cloudy eyes towards the window. 'As I prepared my sermons, I could hear her laughter and Tess merrily barking in the garden. The garden . . .' he sighed again. 'I'm afraid I've let that go. In fact, I've let most things go.'

There was an uneasy silence as the Reverend Gladstone studied the backs of his scrawny hands, while I continued to stroke Tess's narrow forehead.

I looked at the pathetic, crumpled old vicar in the armchair and knew I was getting involved. But after all, I reasoned, it was an old dog and what I was about to do was both practical and humane. Then I looked up at the old man again, the old man whose last link with his dear, departed wife and those happy, carefree days I was about to sever, and I realised there was far more to being a country vet than I had ever imagined.

He pressed his hands onto the arms of the chair, as if he was going to rise, but didn't.

'When my wife suffered so much pain in those last few weeks,' he said softly, 'there were times when I questioned my faith and wondered why it was all so necessary. At least, with Tess, I can repay her loyalty by not letting her linger.'

'Would you like to stay?' I asked.

He shook his head, then moved from the chair to kneel beside me. Shakily he bent forward and cradled the old Setter's head in his arms.

'Remember blackberry time, those warm, easeful days. We'd look for Molly in the fields; you'd see her first, old girl. She'd call and off you'd go, leaping across the stubble to her. Then I would catch you up and take her basket; then home we'd come, all three of us together.' He closed his eyes and pulled the old dog to him. 'Run on now, my Tess, to dear Molly. And I'll be with you shortly.'

He grabbed my arm as he rose and for a few seconds, head bowed, hung on to me. Then looking up, eyes tearful but still set with a gentle smile, he said:

'I'll leave her in your care, young man.' Then he shuffled to the door and drew it and the sagging curtain closed behind him.

I stood for a few seconds looking at her; I was full up and my eyes were feeling gritty, so I took a deep breath and opened the case.

Tess looked up momentarily as the fine needle entered her vein; then, as the barbiturate flooded her bloodstream, her breathing quickened slightly, she took two deeper breaths and lowered her head back onto her paws, as if she was very tired. Then she was still. Tess was dead, and I had killed her.

I pulled the patchwork blanket across and put the syringe and bottle away. After a few minutes I called the Reverend Gladstone; he offered me a sherry, but his hand shook so much that most of it spilled upon the floor. I asked if he would like me to take Tess away, but he declined, saying he would bury her in the garden. Then he walked with me to the gate and, as we parted, even asked God to bless me.

Half a mile out of Brentdor, I stopped on a grassy sward just off the road and sat for quite some time, just thinking.

*   *   *

'All work and no play makes Hubert a dull vet!' observed Charlie on the Tuesday evening of my last week. 'You'll be leaving soon and we haven't had a night out together, yet. Well, social that is,' he added, rubbing his hands eagerly. 'Mind you, some of those calls have been a bit of a lark, I'll give you that.' For having whetted Charlie's veterinary appetite at the Ridways', he had since joined me on several night visits and, as the territory was still rather foreign to me, his company was welcome and also reassuring, especially as I had managed to persuade him to tone down his 'gear' for our rural expeditions.

'How about a jar at the Ravens tonight?' he suggested. 'Promised you a knees-up there, didn' I? Tell your guvnor your going to look at a "leedle Frog pooch".' He pointed to the phone.

It was true that, so far, my time at Ledingford had seemed all work with little opportunity for relaxation, my only diversions being an evening when Brad had invited me to a talk on Australia at Putsley Church Hall and a visit to the cinema to see a Western, during which I fell fast asleep. A 'knees-up' was due, I concluded.

'Good idea!' I told Charlie. 'I'll give Bob Hacker a ring.'

Bob sounded in an unusually good mood and agreed to handle anything that came in, so after a wash and brush up I was ready to go.

'Have a nice time,' said Brad, though her expression changed to one of mild disapproval when she learned where we were going.

The Three Ravens Club was established in a large country house on the outskirts of the town. The old residence had obviously seen more genteel times, but was now given over to the demands of the modern clientele. Although it was termed a club, the rules seemed very flexible, for when Charlie explained that when we got there, he would sign me in, I enquired how long he had been a member. But he just tapped his nose, in the manner of C. J. Pink, and replied that he wasn't.

There were several cars parked on the gravel forecourt and I pulled up the little Ford on the end of the line. Charlie was out before I could secure the brake.

'Come on, Hubert!' he shouted. 'We're wasting good drinking time.'

I followed up the steps to the extensive porch, supported by columns in the Grecian style, not unlike those outside the Merchants Hall but smaller, chipped and in need of restoration. In fact, the whole place appeared a bit run down, although inside the lights were bright and, even with the door closed, I could hear the strains of lively music.

The interior hallway was lit by a showy chandelier which, together with the heavily embossed plum-coloured wallpaper, was obviously designed to give the impression of unashamed luxury, but didn't quite get away with it. There were several archways leading off into side rooms. I caught sight of a gaming table in one, and there was a card school in progress in another. Charlie led off confidently down a long passage and we eventually emerged into an oak-panelled bar.

''Allo, Charlie!'

The voice was unmistakable.

''Allo, Mimi!' mimicked Charlie. 'Look 'oo I 'ave brought for you.' And standing to one side, with a wide sweep of his arm, he presented me to Mimi Lafont who was in attendance behind the counter. She was visible only from the waist upwards, a factor that accentuated her positives in no uncertain manner. Yet as soon as my eyes had re-coordinated themselves, my nostrils were being titillated by the delights of her exotic perfume. She wore a pink, diaphanous blouse abundant with frills and, lodged in the 'V' of the extremely low neck was that rose, the one whose presence absolved the garment, but barely in the nick of time, of any degree of impropriety.

I smiled and nodded at the delicious creature.

'Mr Lasgarn,' she cooed. ''Ow lovely.' Then she gave a

sideways glance and, touching her lips briefly with the back of her jewelled hand, said coyly:

'Now I 'ave two of you. 'Ow lovely.'

I followed her glance to the end of the bar where, seated on a high stool with a large whisky before him, was none other than McBean.

'Well now, Hugh,' he acknowledged, 'now there's a surprise an' all. You'll be here for the experience, I shouldn't wonder?'

'You might say that,' I countered, copying Charlie's style. 'And then again — you might not.'

Charlie appeared bemused by the banter, so I introduced him to my colleague.

After handshakes and greetings, McBean ordered two pints, took another whisky for himself and Mimi joined us with a port and lemon.

Charlie was soon rabbiting on about a trip he had once made to Ireland, and how he hadn't enjoyed it because 'it rained all the bleedin' time' and he had difficulty in understanding the 'lingo'. McBean listened tolerantly until Charlie said:

'No wonder all Micks are little, it's gettin' wet all the time. Shrinks 'em, you see.' He raised his glass and called, 'Cheerio.' I could see McBean was becoming irritated, so I changed the subject and enquired of Mimi how Petal was faring.

'She still 'as a leedle trouble,' she replied, flashing her lashes. 'But with you and "Iggy" to look after her, I know she will be wonderfool!'

'Iggy!' I repeated.

'Ignatius,' she explained, casting an alluring glance at McBean.

McBean coughed, said, 'Well now,' and finished his whisky. This revelation gave another dimension to McBean's character, for surprisingly enough, in my three weeks at Hacker's, I had never thought of him as other than Mr McBean, McBean or just Mac — or on such close terms with Mimi Lafont, either.

It was Charlie who, putting his glass back upon the counter, couldn't resist following up the line. 'Another whisky, Iggy?' he asked, his face showing not the slightest trace of flippancy.

McBean nodded, but I could see in his eyes that he wasn't taking too kindly to my Cockney companion.

We sat drinking for some time, Charlie doing most of the talking, while Mimi occasionally detached herself to attend to other members in the bar. Charlie had got to the point where he was displaying his expertise at bar tricks with piles of pennies, when McBean asked: 'Ever seen a "whisky knock", Charlie?'

Charlie eyed McBean suspiciously and slowly shook his head, then his face gradually broke into a smile as he realised there could well be some catch in the question.

'Come on, let's have it,' he said. 'What's a "whisky knock"?'

'Now there's a thing, Hugh,' said McBean. But we couldn't really expect a gentleman from the City to know, could we?' Then, turning to Mimi, he asked for a whisky. 'In one of those wee glasses, there.' He pointed to a row of small goblets. 'And some ginger ale, if you please.'

With the requirements before him, McBean assumed the pose of a conjuror by raising his arms so that his jacket sleeves fell back slightly, as if to demonstrate that all was above board and he had nothing concealed about his person.

Charlie watched with undivided attention.

First, McBean held up the goblet and appraised its contents; then, after replacing it upon the counter, he dipped the end of his forefinger into the amber liquid and moistened the rim of the glass with a circular motion. Finally, he touched the end of his tongue with his finger-tip, to avoid any wastage.

'Now watch carefully,' he said, slowly and deliberately. 'This must be done very quickly.'

For a few seconds he sat poised with his hands held over the drink; then, taking a deep breath, he shot into action.

Grabbing the ginger ale, he topped up the scotch with the left hand, covering the glass immediately afterwards with the palm of his right. Then, ale bottle down, he took the goblet in his left hand, still covered with the right, thumped it hard on his knee, uncovered the glass and downed it in one.

'There!' he announced smugly, smoothing his dampened moustache down at each side. 'That's a "whisky knock".'

'So what!' exclaimed Charlie, turning to me with an expression of amused bewilderment upon his face.

'Let's see you do it,' challenged McBean.

Charlie slapped his knee. 'You're a mad Mick and no mistake,' he roared.

'A little wager,' added McBean. 'Five bob ye can't.'

'Five bob I can't!' Charlie dissolved in laughter, but on recovering, he dug his hand deep into his powder-blue drainpipe pocket and slapped two halfcrowns on the counter.

'You're on, Iggy! You're on!' he shouted. 'Set 'em up, darlin'.'

Mimi obliged and Charlie went through the ritual step by step as demonstrated by McBean: first appraising the whisky, then moistening the rim and licking his forefinger. When all set, he turned to the assembled company that had now grown to a small group as other members were drawn with interest to the contest.

'Now you all watch very carefully. I've got to be quick, so I have, an' all, an' all,' Charlie announced in a mock Irish accent and, taking a deep breath as McBean had done, he was off. In went the ginger ale, then swiftly he covered the glass with his palm. Snatching it from the counter with his free hand, he thumped it violently on his knee and raised the glass to his lips.

But, as he took his right hand away to drink, the effervescing contents foamed up instantaneously, exploding in his face, leaving him dripping in a bubbly mix of whisky and ginger ale.

Charlie spluttered and wrung his hands amid the laughter.

'My God!' he exclaimed. 'Even my bleedin' pants are soaked!'

'Well, now, Charlie me boy,' commented McBean, as he reverently removed the two halfcrowns from the counter, 'at least Micks only get wet in the rain!'

Charlie, however, took it all in good part. 'All right. Where did I go wrong?' he asked, unbuttoning his shirt to mop up with a large handkerchief.

'Buy me another whisky and I'll show you,' said McBean, at which point Charlie realised his opponent had got him very much over a barrel and, with a broad smile, held out a hand and said: 'Iggy, my son. I'll give you best!'

At that moment a rather overdressed, middle-aged blonde came into the bar and called: 'Mr Lasgarn here?' Seeing me acknowledge, she said, 'Telephone for you. At the desk.'

'You're not on call?' asked McBean.

'Didn't think so,' I said, slipping from my stool. 'Bob Hacker said he'd handle things.'

I followed the overdressed female to the small reception kiosk. She handed the phone across the counter and attempted to assume a disinterest in my caller, by re-arranging an already neat display of leaflets in a holder on the wall.

'It's Percy, Mr Lasgarn. He's had an accident. Could you come home, please!' It was Brad, sounding terribly distressed. 'He's in the kitchen . . .' Her voice faltered and I could tell she was crying. 'He's just crawled in, bleeding and in an awful state. Please come home!'

'Brad, I'll be there straight away,' I said. 'Don't worry. I'm coming now.' I heard her give a sniff, then she put the phone down.

'Everything all right?' enquired the overdressed blonde.

'Percy's had an accident,' I replied.

'Relative?' she asked.

'No,' I said, 'a friend. Just a friend.' Then I made my way

172

hastily back to the bar.

'I'm going back to the digs, now,' I told my drinking companions.

'I'll come with you,' offered Charlie, rising from his stool.

'No need,' I said. 'I can manage.'

'So you might,' he replied, shaking his sticky trousers. 'But Percy's a mate of mine. Come on.'

'Want any help?' asked McBean.

'Don't know yet,' I admitted. 'But it doesn't sound too good.'

'Ring back if you do. 9730, isn't it?' He turned to Mimi.

'Yes,' she said. 'Good luck.'

Percy was lying in his favourite spot by the stove in the kitchen. Brad had covered him with a woollen blanket.

'He hasn't moved since he came in,' she sobbed, gathering the collar of her dressing gown closer.

I carefully drew back the blanket to reveal Percy lying on his right side. He raised his head slightly in response to my movement, but it obviously caused him pain and he unsteadily lowered it again. Sticky, bloodstained saliva covered his face, his tongue protruding slightly over a sagging lower jaw.

'Will he be all right?' asked Brad tearfully.

'Don't you worry, m'dear.' Charlie put his arm tenderly around her shoulders. 'Hugh here will fix him, if anybody can.'

I paid no apparent heed to the compliment, though secretly I was very flattered and only hoped I could come up to Charlie's expectations. He himself was certainly very concerned and upset, which had probably accounted for him calling me Hugh, for the very first time.

I lifted Percy up and motioned to Charlie to put the blanket on the table, then gently I laid the poor creature on it and commenced my examination.

'Could you fetch my case from the car, Charlie?' He nodded and disappeared.

From the colour of the membranes around the eyes, I deduced that Percy had not lost an excessive amount of blood, despite the haemorrhage from the mouth. There were no broken limbs, no scars or abrasions on his skin, but his coat on the left side was contaminated with what appeared to be red sand. Charlie returned with the case and opened it ready for me to use.

With my stethoscope I listened to Percy's chest; the breathing was shallow but regular and his heart steady. There was no evidence of broken ribs or lung damage.

'So far, so good,' I commented.

'Car accident?' asked Charlie.

'Could be,' I agreed. Then, cautiously I opened Percy's mouth. As I did so, he tensed and dug his claws deeply into the fabric of the woollen blanket, at the same time giving a low growl of anguish. But for me, one glimpse was enough to recognise that his jaw had been broken; the teeth on the right side were displaced at least half an inch above those opposite.

'That hurt him!' exclaimed Charlie, wincing as if experiencing the pain personally. 'What is it?'

'Fractured jaw,' I replied. 'Right at the symphisis — the join,' I explained. 'At the front.'

'Oh!' gasped Brad. 'Poor Percy. Don't put him to sleep. Please!'

'Can you do anything?' Charlie's face was quite white. 'Anything at all?'

'It's a nasty one,' I admitted. 'He's had a crack on the jaw, all right. Trouble is, fixing it so that he will still be able to eat. You can't plaster that area.'

I moistened some cotton wool and cleaned Percy's face. He seemed to appreciate my attention, closing his eyes and slightly raising his aching head as if trying to assist in any way he could. I thought of the evenings when he would relax on the chair in front of me — not a care in the world. And now this. Poor old chap.

Suddenly I knew I was becoming involved again. How difficult it was to be detached, I thought, yet I had to be.

For if I could do nothing, I would have to put Percy down and that would be heartbreaking for Brad — and Charlie — and, I had to admit it, for me as well.

'It wants a brace,' I said, thinking aloud. 'Like a wire brace.' If I could fix the jawbones together with wire, it would still allow the tongue to function and Percy could at least lap. 'It wants to be fairly fine and strong, but pliable.'

'Like fuse wire,' said Charlie.

'Fuse wire?'

'Yea, thick fuse wire. Wind it round his cutters — what d'you call them?'

'Carnacials,' I said thoughtfully. 'Yes, that could work. Brad, have you got any?'

Brad, who seemed to have composed herself, ferreted about in a kitchen drawer and eventually held up a card.

'Thirty-amp should do the trick,' I said, studying it. 'But I'll have to put Percy out first.'

Over the next half hour, with Charlie's assistance and Brad hovering about in the background, I anaesthetised Percy with a barbiturate injection and, after cleaning up the jaw, secured the fractured ends in place with the fuse wire. To ensure that the brace wouldn't slip, I had to pass the free ends through the skin flaps of his lower jaw to meet in a twist under his chin. Finally, I dressed my handiwork with some antiseptic ointment.

'Nice bit of engineering, Hubert,' said Charlie, as I washed up. 'Ole Percy will think he's done ten rounds with Joe Erskine when he wakes up.'

'He will wake up?' asked Brad anxiously.

'Yes, I'm sure he will,' I said. 'Percy's a tough old stick, he'll make it. He'll obviously have a bit of difficulty eating at first, so milk with sugar or Bovril would be a good starter.'

The clatter of the door knocker broke abruptly into our conversation.

'Now who could that be, at this time of night?' said Brad, a trifle nervously.

'I'll go,' said Charlie. 'Could be the *News of the World* come to get my story!'

I heard greetings and laughter, then McBean popped his head round the door.

'Well now,' he began, 'I was just running Mimi — Miss Lafont — home and I thought I'd call by to see what was afoot.'

By the exotic aroma that wafted after him I deduced that Mimi — Miss Lafont — was not very far behind. Sure enough, she was there and I could hear Charlie introducing her to Brad in the hallway. I explained the circumstances to McBean who carefully scrutinised Percy's repaired jaw before standing back and after a cursory smoothing of his moustache, pronouncing judgement.

'Good bit of work, Hugh, good bit of work,' he commented. 'Seen this type o' thing once or twice before. It's usually caused by a fall, cat jumping for a wall and misjudging the distance. Cracks his chin and splits the symphisis.'

'That's how he did it,' said Brad who had overheard McBean's comments. 'You silly boy,' she scolded, though Percy was quite oblivious of the reprimand, being still deeply asleep. 'Some nights,' she explained, 'if he's shut out, he climbs the apple tree and jumps onto my window sill.'

'That explains the sand on his coat,' I added. 'The builders left a pile on the concrete below.'

'Well, Mimi,' said Charlie, 'hope it's not so dangerous getting into your bedroom.'

'Charlie!' exploded Mimi, patting the air with her hand, as she usually did when pretending to be disapproving, but enjoying it really.

Brad, with a look of slight embarrassment, suggested that she make some cocoa.

'How long do you think the brace should stay on?' I asked McBean.

'About a month should do it,' he replied.

'Will you see to taking it off?' I asked.

'Me?' he questioned.

'I can't,' I explained. 'I'll be finished here next week.'

'Well now!' McBean took my arm and secretively turned me into the corner, facing the saucepan rack and bread bin. 'Bob and I have been talking,' he confided. 'You see, now that his father is dead, we're going to be a bit short-handed. And I think we could get a deferment for you from the Army, for a while anyway, if you'd like to stay. It's up to you, of course. It's not so bad here, and — well now —' he assumed a very dour expression, as if he was about to say something very profound. '— I'd like you to stay, if you would. Think it over.'

The offer took me completely by surprise. I thanked him for it and said I would consider the suggestion. Brad was busying herself with cups and saucers, and through in the hallway I could see Charlie offering to listen to Mimi's heart with my stethoscope. Percy was still relaxed, but gradually starting to come around.

It was a good offer, but was I just putting off the inevitable National Service? Perhaps it would be better to get it over. Yet I was happy at Ledingford, and who was to say if there would be a job available here again?

'Cocoa's ready,' said Brad. And as I followed her into the dining room, she turned and said, 'Percy and I would like you to stay, too.'

Seven

The following morning I was unable to discuss with Bob Hacker the opportunity of extending my stay in Ledingford, as both he and McBean had taken early calls. I had been left the job of dehorning a small herd of dairy cows at Redwarden, so there was ample time to deliberate my immediate future as I trundled along the Brecon Road.

Even if I elected to stay, I still could not be absolutely sure that I would qualify for deferment. McBean had said that there had been talk of National Service being abandoned, but that was not definite either, and I did not fancy spending the coming months in an atmosphere of uncertainty. Of course, in the Royal Army Veterinary Corps I would be eligible for a commission on entry, because of my degree. Captain Lasgarn sounded pretty good and an officer's life had a lot going for it. Army vets were posted all over the world; the chance to travel at Her Majesty's expense was something to be seriously considered. All in all, it was not an easy decision.

However, as I swung off the main road and turned down towards the river, I decided to concentrate on the job in hand — the unsavoury business of chopping the horns off cattle.

It was to be the first time that I would carry out the procedure all by myself. Previously I had watched demonstrations in my final student year and been part of a group in the practical course which had removed the elegant but lethal appendages from a herd of Ayrshires.

Lethal indeed they were — long, curved and sharp as lances — and it was their destructive potential, acceptable in the wild but prohibitive under housed conditions, that was the reason for their removal.

Punctured udders, ripped flanks and damaged eyes were some of the many injuries caused by spiteful or aggressive horned cows, and a 'boss' with sharp horns could wreak havoc, if she so had a mind.

In fact, only six months previously, a veterinary surgeon had unfortunately been killed while carrying out a Ministry Tuberculin Test. The poor chap had been standing beside the neck of an Ayrshire cow, about to measure her skin reaction. As he stooped to read the size on the calipers, she threw her head back and, such was the length and curvature of her horns, that it fractured his skull and he died almost immediately.

So, while the dehorning procedure appeared barbaric to some folk, there were very practical and humane reasons why it was carried out.

In Glasgow, the cows had been given general anaesthesia by placing a chloroform mask over their heads. In a few minutes they would collapse and the horns were sawn off at the butt, any haemorrhage being stemmed with hot irons. They were soon coming round and standing up, appearing none the worse, and the wounds would heal well within a few weeks. It was quite amusing to watch them afterwards, still holding their heads very carefully when passing through narrow doorways, not realising that their horns were gone and that negotiating such obstacles was now much easier.

There was one major snag with the general anaesthesia method: cattle are not, at any time, good subjects for complete sedation, due to the reaction of their large stomachs. These, when in a relaxed condition, can allow gas to accumulate to such an extent that the resultant tympany presses upon the chest cavity, impeding the action of heart and lungs, sometimes with fatal consequences.

'You are liable to lose one cow in two hundred, with this method,' the demonstrator had told us — which he thought was reasonably acceptable. I remember thinking at the time, how tough if it was the first one and how difficult it would be to retain the farmer's confidence by proclaiming that the next one hundred and ninety-nine would be perfectly all right.

The method used in the Hacker practice was harder but safer, for the cow, anyway. Local anaesthetic was used to block the nerves to the horns, and separation was achieved by the use of massive shears that had long iron handles connected to a rachet operating razor-sharp steel blades. The whole apparatus was extremely unwieldy and quite heavy, and with the cow still conscious and often very active, even though her horns were frozen, it was a very physical job, to say the least.

The directions I had been given were that, after crossing the narrow brick bridge over the river at Redwarden, I was to take the road that led to the right of the Red Lion and follow it up the hill. As I rounded the sharp bend at the side of the pub, I was confronted with what appeared to be a vertical ascent, and such was the tightness of the curved approach that I lost momentum. The Ford had only three forward gears, the first necessitating momentary stoppage of the vehicle — not being 'synchromesh', as I was informed on receiving my transport. This, I had discovered, could be quite hair-raising when on a gradient, and the risk of running backwards very real, the brakes not being of any great efficiency, especially in reverse.

Just at the point where I executed my change into first, I noticed, standing nearby, a roadman, old and bent, with battered trilby, rolled-up sleeves, waistcoat sporting a dangling Albert, moleskins tied below the knee and clumpy boots.

'Steep, isn't it!' I called. He leaned on his spade, took his pipe from his mouth, nodded, then spat — but before he could speak, I was away, grinding up the hill.

I sat perfectly still, just fingertips touching the steering and, as the pitch increased, I leaned forward, moving my bottom to the extreme edge of the seat in an attempt to give my mount every assistance. The road ahead appeared like a wall and was getting steeper by every yard, and the engine was labouring as I had never known it before. There was a smell, too, acrid and burning, and suddenly, with a groan of anguish, she died and I started to run back jerkily — the little Ford was beaten.

I jammed on the brakes and realised that I would have to run down backwards, which I gradually did, my heart in my mouth.

At the bottom, the old roadman was waiting.

'She wouldn't have it,' I said. 'I'll have another run.'

He nodded understandingly but made no comment, and I suspected that my type of predicament was nothing new to him.

The next attempt got me just a few yards farther up the hill before defeat sent me running down again.

This time, the old boy offered some advice.

'Too much weight on!' he shouted from the verge.

He could well be right, I thought, for the dehorning shears were certainly heavy, but they had to stay, because they were essential to my visit.

'Can I leave some boxes here until I come back?' I asked.

He nodded, so I off-loaded as much kit as I thought I wouldn't need and left it at the roadside, asking the old man if he'd keep an eye on it. Then I set to and attacked for the third time.

It was better by another ten yards, but still nowhere near the summit. I pulled the brake and rested precariously on the gradient, wondering if I dared get out and deposit the shears, then have a fresh run and, if I made it, walk back down and pick them up. The other alternative was first to carry them all the way up, then come back for the car — but I didn't fancy that.

Back to the bottom of the hill I went yet again, and this time the old roadman put down his spade and came across to the window.

'I 'ad a mare once,' he said. 'Good looker and strong, but the mind of a woman. Could be sweet as a buttercup one day and a devil the next. Would never lead into the stable, no matter what I did. Coax 'er, put feed in the manger, beat 'er — she wouldn' go.' He paused and stood back from the window.

'So, how did you get her in?' I asked, knowing full well what was expected of me.

He drew on his pipe, then spat and came closer again and, with a twinkle in his eye, said: 'I backed 'er in. Now, you turn about, young fella, an' back 'er up. 'Er'll go!'

And sure enough, I turned round and went up the hill backwards to the very top.

When eventually I got onto the flat, I stopped. The lower reverse gear ratio and redistribution of weight had done it, but, despite my university degree, I had to admit that it had taken a little old countryman to tell me.

The dehorning was rough, despite the fact that Seth Owen, the farmer, had two strong sons to help. The main problem was that the cows were not very accessible, being chained in stalls in three low, dark houses.

Firstly, I went through them with the injection of local anaesthetic, putting a small dose under the skin along the ridge below each horn, to freeze the cornual nerves. The Owen boys were strong and held the cows' heads firmly, one hand in the nose and the other on the horn — but I was hard put to see properly and twice injected my finger. To prevent haemorrhage, I tied binder twine in a figure of eight around the poll at the butt of the horns, as suggested by Bob Hacker. This had a tourniquet effect and could be removed in a few days when the wound was healing. A light dressing of sulphonamide powder on the cut stump was the only other requirement.

It took about three-quarters of an hour and, after getting squeezed, kicked, trodden upon and self-injected, I was ready for the amputation.

One Owen son steadied the first cow's head whilst I raised the mighty choppers and placed the blades at the base of the horns. The handles of the infernal machine were so splayed that the younger Owen and I had to stretch our arms wide to reach. The confined space made the whole exercise extremely awkward and the contortions we were forced to assume were mind-boggling. When suitably positioned, we pulled the handles and, with a sickening crunch, the horn was severed.

Younger horns came away easily because they were mostly hollow, but with age, they became solid and snapped through rather than cut. Several times I unfortunately placed the shears too low and cut the strings, so that the tourniquet was broken and thin streams of blood spurted everywhere, covering my face and arms so that I was bloody, sweaty, sore and getting progressively fed up.

The last cow was an old, grey Shorthorn with wickedly inward-curving horns the colour of ivory. There was a country theory that, by counting the annular ridges on a horn and adding two, one could estimate the bearer's age — but on Gert, for such was her title, the rings were so tightly knit and so numerous, that they were impossible to count.

'This is the one we've been waiting for,' voiced Seth, as we started on our final chop. And if he'd been waiting for her, considering that all he had done was to stand back and give advice, my delight at seeing the end to the gory task was unquantifiable.

After placing the shears with some difficulty over the horn, the younger Owen and I took the strain. Previously, two heaves at the most had been sufficient, but four heaves later and the blades had hardly nibbled at Gert's formidable antlers. Young Owen and I heaved and jerked in all postures until, finally, Seth said: 'I'll give yer a pound.'

Coming behind us he grabbed the handles, but his weight caused the shears to twist so that the right metal handle on which we were pulling, came directly above my head.

Suddenly, there was a mighty 'CRACK' and I felt the horn give, followed by a hollow ringing in my head and my knees collapsing.

I was aware of a small waterfall cascading down my spine — there was music, too, and pain — shooting pain between my eyes. I found myself in a crouched position on the cobbles outside the cowhouse, whither the Owens had carried me. Seth had poured cold water over me — hence the cascading sensation — and as I opened my eyes I dimly glimpsed the three of them, standing together in a blue haze, looking down upon me.

'You all right?' enquired Seth, poised with half a bucket left in case I wasn't.

My hand strayed to my forehead.

'Proper goose egg you got there,' said the younger Owen. 'Knocked you for six, it did.'

'Knocked me for six, indeed.' And as I slumped there, on the cobbles, my head thumping, clothes soaking wet, my body in a cold sweat and covered in blood, part mine, part Seth's cows', I decided that Army life would be a holiday compared to country practice.

*   *   *

Bob Hacker was disappointed when I told him I was not intending to stay on at Ledingford.

'Think it over, Hugh. Don't let a crack on the head distort your vision,' he said, laughingly. 'You've settled in well and we really could do with you. Anyway, you don't have to let me know until Friday, so just say you'll think it over, eh?'

I agreed to do just that. The dehorning episode certainly wasn't the main reason for my decision against staying, though it may just have tipped the balance. Neither was it any patriotic urge to join the Army. No, the real reason, which I knew lay deep inside my mind, was that I was coming to love the countryside, the farming, the livestock and the way of life, so much that, the deeper my roots went down, the less I should want to leave and the greater the final wrench when the time came — as, inevitably, it would.

Work finished early and I was back in the digs by four o'clock. Brad was more than sympathetic over the lump on my head and insisted on making me submit to a witch hazel compress which, to my surprise and relief, worked wonders by taking much of the soreness from my head. Although the comfort that she bestowed was somewhat diminished by her relating to me how dangerous blows to the head could be, and how a man she once knew, after suffering a similar contusion, whilst appearing to recover well, died three days later from a 'clot' on the brain.

Just after six, McBean rang.

'Still alive, Hugh!' he chuckled, which remark, coupled with Brad's reminiscences, did not find immediate favour with me. 'Fancy a party tonight?' he continued. 'Do you good. Just a casual get-together out at Stokley. Pam Sangston is giving it. London girl, but comes down to stay with her aunt quite a bit. You'll meet some of the young blood and the talent is usually quite presentable. What d'ye say, now?'

I had intended to feel ill and suffer that evening, as physically I was sore and mentally browned off.

McBean sensed my indecision.

'Come on, man. You don't want to die a recluse, do ye now!' he chided.

'Oh, God! I thought, death again. And if, according to Brad, it could come in three days, I'd best enjoy what was left.

'Thanks, Mac. I'd like to come,' I answered.

'Good for you,' he replied heartily. 'Pick ye up at eight!'

After a bath, a shave, a change of clothes and a meal, I felt a great deal better and began looking forward to the evening. I would be meeting people of my own age group, which was something that I had missed from university life. It was going to be good.

At ten to eight, McBean rang to say he couldn't make it.

'Well, now, not until much later, that is,' he explained. 'There's a calving at Hecton. You go ahead, Pam knows that you're coming. As a matter of fact,' he added, 'she asked me to bring you!' He spilled out the directions to Stokley; about two miles beyond the village, I was to turn left at some white railings and the house would be the first that I came too.

Suddenly, I didn't feel so keen, but again McBean's Irish intuition came into play. 'Now, you will go, Hugh, won't you!' he insisted and I agreed that I would.

'Good,' he said. 'I'll be along as soon as I can, just tell Pam why I shall be late, there's a good chap. See you, Hugh . . .' and with that, he cleared the line.

I arrived at my destination just on nine o'clock.

It was an attractive half-timbered house set back a little way from the road, and might well have been a small farmhouse at one time, for there were several small but well-maintained buildings ranged around a gravelled yard. There were about seven cars in all, practically filling the free space, but I managed to squeeze in between a large Wolseley and a smart open-top MG.

Leaving my duffle in the car, I approached the house. Heavily lined curtains covered all the windows, but the chinks of light filtering through the gaps indicated that practically every room was lit, even upstairs as well. An ancient porch led to a formidable, studded oak door with a black iron ring for the knocker, with which I announced my presence.

Eventually the door was opened by a slim, dark-haired girl in a lime-green taffeta dress, whom I assumed was Pam Sangston. I explained who I was and why I had arrived alone, and presented McBean's apologies. All the time I was talking, she looked at me very intently with her large brown eyes. When I had concluded my introduction, she stepped forward and kissed me on the cheek.

'How super!' she said, grabbing my arm. 'Come and meet everybody.'

But despite my attractive hostess's invitation and enthusiasm, what happened next proved somewhat of an anticlimax.

Pam led me into a long, lowbeamed room full of sombre, black oak furniture. A reasonably hospitable fire flickered in the hearth, but that appeared to be the only noticeably spontaneous movement. There must have been a dozen or so young people seated around the perimeter: large, roundfaced, solemn-looking lads on the right, grasping beer glasses; girls on the left, four of them squeezed together on a brown hide settee, one in an armchair and the other on a piano stool. The quartet on the settee were all gigglers, the one in the armchair, ginger with freckles; but the blonde on the piano stool looked rather nice.

'This is Hugh Lasgarn — he's a vet,' announced Pam gaily, holding up my arm, rather like a referee at a boxing contest.

'Isn't Iggy McBean coming?' asked one of the girls on the settee.

'No, he's gone to see a cow,' I said, trying to sound as relaxed and casual as I felt able.

'Gone to see a cow,' repeated the girl in the armchair. 'I wonder what her name is!' With that, the four on the settee burst into fits of laughter and began slapping each other's knees in their hilarity.

Pam appeared slightly embarrassed.

'I don't suppose you know everybody,' she said, which was rather a kind way of expressing the fact that I didn't know anybody. 'I'll go round this way,' she announced, starting with the boys. There were a couple of Johns, a Dudley, a Graham, a Philip and a Frank, and a tall lad, the only one who got up and shook hands, called Raymond — the rest just nodded and drank their beer. Then, it was Polly in the armchair, a Jane, a Margaret, a Felicity and another Jane on the settee, who all said 'Hullo' together and then set off on another mass giggle. Diana on the piano stool gave me a gracious smile and said, 'How do you do, Hugh,' at which I marked her down as the most attractive bird there.

'Get Hugh a beer, John,' said Pam.

The two Johns rose, then sat down again, each expecting the other to get it, then the tall youth, Raymond, got up and fetched a bottle of Cheltenham and Gloucester Pale Ale from another room. Then there was a knock on the door and Pam went away to greet some other guests.

I took a seat and started to chat, but it was tough going all the way. The conversation was of the simple question and answer type, but I learned about the price of lambs, why some tractors were difficult to start in the cold, who would win the Stock Judging Cup and why the pheasants were 'thin on the ground'. Then Dudley went out and returned with a case of Cheltenham and Gloucester which he set on the floor before us and this thoughtful act seemed to ease the tension; the conversation turned to Rugby, and at last I began to enjoy the evening.

Meanwhile, the girls had disappeared and strains of music wafted from another room — 'The Saints Go Marching In', 'The Tender Trap' and other pop tunes. Pam came through on two occasions ordering us to go and dance, but nobody seemed very keen. Then she called us to eat and the company rose as one man and made for the kitchen.

The table took my breath away, for there was turkey, ham and a great cut of roast beef surrounded by pies, sausages, chutneys and cheese. The side table was laden with sweets and trifles and mouthwatering gâteaux — such a feast I hadn't seen before. The atmosphere was now one of jollity and fun as plates were piled high, glasses filled and everyone set to and ate their fill.

When all were suitably replete and rested, the dancing started again and I was collared by the ginger Polly. She was 'comfortable' to say the least, but when someone, by design or accident, put out the lights, she turned into a clockwork limpet and my body experienced degrees of compression that it had never known before. It made the morning's rough-up at Seth Owen's seem like light exercise; my opinion of the area as a rural backwater, and any preconceived ideas I had of the naivety of country girls, were stood firmly upon their heads.

After that passionate encounter, I danced with Pam in a pleasant but more sedate fashion and then with one of the Janes, but I couldn't seem to get near the blonde, who was persistently monopolised by one of the Johns.

I joined a 'spoof' school which had been set up by the boys. It consisted of guessing who had how many coins in a closed hand, betting on the results. It was a new game to me and I lost twelve shillings. Then came a competition of walking on beer bottles, a feat of which I had considerable experience from my Glasgow days. A line was drawn and, with feet behind it, the participant stretched forward supported by two Cheltenham and Gloucesters, one in each hand. The object was to leave one bottle as far forward as possible, returning in backward hops, both hands on the remaining bottle, without collapsing on the floor.

My main opponent was the John who was with the blonde Diana, and I was determined to beat him. But he must have had a bit of practice, for he left his bottle two inches beyond my best attempt and in trying to beat it, I slipped, hitting my head upon the floor and revitalising the painful lump which, until then, I had completely forgotten.

At that moment I lost my spirit of fair play and resented my victor, not only for his monopoly of the most attractive girl in the room, but for beating me at the bottles, at which I was normally invincible.

'Doesn't look as if McBean is coming,' commented Raymond, as we sat together in a corner after the contest.

'Probably finished too late,' I suggested.

'No point wasting his beer,' said Raymond, handing me another bottle, and we settled into a quiet little session together.

It as well past midnight when the first guests started to leave, and I decided that I should make a move as well. I was seeking out Pam, to thank her for the evening, and trying to avoid Polly who kept crossing my path rather obviously, when the larger John came in through the front door.

'Ah, Hugh. You going back to Ledingford?' he asked.

'Yes,' I said. 'Why?'

'Could you give my girl a lift. Damned car won't fire — and she has to get back. Pam says we could stay here, but she won't have it.' He winked.

'Of course, John,' I replied. 'Yes, of course. No trouble!'

'Aha,' I thought. Things were looking up, so I speedily found Pam, thanked her and quickly got out to my car. Diana was standing by the MG with a face like thunder.

'Hugh Lasgarn will run you back,' said John. 'Sure you won't stay?'

'No, thank you!' she responded firmly, and tugged her coat around her.

I scuttled to the passenger door and found it locked, so I had to run around to the other side, open the door and lean across. In my haste I hit my head on the roof sill, but I hardly noticed it. Then I scrabbled to clear the seat of my barnacles, two mucklets, a rope and four or five bottles, slinging it all onto the back seat. Finally, after a cursory dusting of the seat with my hand, I opened the door.

But Diana was not standing on ceremony. She got in and sat down, nearly squashing my hand and slammed the passenger door behind her.

'Blasted points!' exclaimed John, 'and now the battery's down. If I leave it half an hour she should kick, but Her Ladyship won't wait.'

'Don't worry,' I replied, 'my pleasure.' And two fingers to you, I thought, for beating me at the bottles.

'Hope yours starts,' he said.

I went cold with fear. At last, the girl on the piano seat to myself and now it all depended on the little Ford. 'Let me down whenever you like,' I murmured. 'Stall on hills, conk out in the middle of nowhere, have four flat tyres and the spare at the same time, but please, please start now!'

I pulled the knob and the engine, all eight horsepower of it, rattled joyously into life.

'You beauty!' I exclaimed, thankfully. 'You little beauty!'

'I beg your pardon!' said Diana, frostily.

'Oh, the car,' I explained. 'I was talking to the car.'

Two locks and I had turned, then, straightening up, headed down the drive to the open road.

'Sorry to put you to all this trouble,' she apologised, as we approached the gateway. 'But John knew very well that I had to be home on time.'

'No trouble at all,' I replied manfully and swung onto the road. It was a tight, right-angled turn and, as I pressed the accelerator to keep momentum, the passenger seat tipped and threw Diana on to me.

'My God! What's happening!' she screamed, her arms folded around my neck. The car lurched and I corrected the swerve, the passenger seat fell back in place and Diana followed it.

'I'd have been safer walking!' She pulled her coat closely about her and stared straight ahead.

'Sorry,' I apologised. 'The seat's loose.'

'That I have discovered,' she retorted icily, and sat in silence as we made for the main road. She didn't speak for about another mile, then she sat up straight and said:

'You're taking me the wrong way!'

'I'm not,' I said, a little annoyed that my navigational skills should be questioned. 'We'll come to Stokley village soon and Ledingford is about nine miles further on.'

'You are taking me the wrong way,' she insisted. 'Now turn around, please!'

I slowed down and pulled up at the side of the road.

'Look, when I came from Ledingford I came through Stokley for about two miles, turned left and got to Pam's. Okay, so coming back I come out of Pam's to the main road, turn right, back through Stokley, which is around the corner, then on to Ledingford.'

'This way leads to Belbury,' Diana said adamantly. 'So please turn round or I'll get out!' She fumbled for the door catch, but couldn't find it. 'Please, Hugh,' she pleaded. 'Turn round.'

So turn round I did. I drove six miles until we came to Belbury, where she apologised, then I turned round again and headed back to Ledingford.

Diana sat in silence, just looking ahead. I gave occasional glances to the side, but it produced no response. The dim dashboard lights were enough for me to see her face and her long, elegant neck. In profile she had a most beautiful face — high cheekbones, fine nose and perfect lips — she really was the most attractive girl I had ever met.

'Won't be long now,' I volunteered, trying to ease the obvious tension. 'Earthquakes and other minor harassments permitting.'

She turned and I glanced to see her smile.

'Sorry I was such a pig, Hugh,' she said, quietly, 'but I was fuming with John and I did think you were taking me the wrong way, honestly!'

A car with its lights full on was rapidly approaching behind, causing me to dip the driving mirror. When it caught up, it hung on my tail for several minutes before making a further move, then it suddenly pulled out and drove alongside.

It was John in his MG.

Even in the semi-darkness, I could discern a vile expression on his face; he shouted something that I couldn't quite hear, but which I guessed was equally vile.

'You know what he's thinking,' I said to Diana, as the tail lights of the MG disappeared in the distance, but by her face, it was obvious she had already realised how John had read the situation.

'Yes,' she replied, frowning. 'I know . . .' Then she put her hand to her lips and started to laugh. 'Serve him right for having such an awful mind.'

For the rest of the journey she chatted away happily. She was a secretary at Seamer's Cider Works. She had no brothers or sisters, liked dancing — particularly Scottish country dancing — cooking and reading, had no pets but wanted a dog. In turn, I gave her a potted history of myself and my career to date, and when I rather hesitantly asked her about the relationship with John, she replied that she had only been out with him a few times, a fact which cheered me considerably.

Eventually we arrived at her home.

'Thank you ever so much, Hugh,' she said, giving me a charming smile. 'It was so kind of you to bring me home. Sorry about those extra miles.'

'Could I see you again?' I asked.

Diana gave a slight gasp, then said, 'But you're finishing this week.'

'Oh, no,' I said, without any hesitation. 'Oh no. I came with the option of leaving if I didn't like it — but no, I shall probably stay on for a little while anyway.'

'Well, there's a Young Farmers' Dance at Beckhampton, next Wednesday. We could go to that if you'd like — they're usually good fun.'

'Grand. What time shall I call for you?'

'About eight.'

'I'll be here.'

'Goodnight, Hugh.' She unlatched the gate and I watched her run to the front door. She turned again and waved, I briefly saw her face in the porch light — then she was gone and the door closed behind her.

I stood for a few moments looking at the house until the porch light went out, thinking to myself how strange it was that a logical, calculated decision could suddenly be made illogical, yet very much more acceptable.

I got back into the car feeling quite light headed — and it wasn't the beer or the crack on my head, which I felt to make sure I was the same person.

'Come on, you little beauty,' I shouted, happily. 'Let's go home.' And the little Ford burst into life, but because of the extra miles, she ran out of petrol at the bottom of Putsley Pitch and I had to leave her and walk.

As I locked the door before leaving, I patted her affectionately on the wing.

'You're still a little beauty,' I told her. 'Thank you very much.'

Bob Hacker appeared pleased, when I told him the following morning that I would like to stay.

'I'll get on to the Ministry right away,' he said, shaking my hand warmly. 'You never know what this might lead to.'

And as blonde hair and blue eyes had suddenly monopolised my thoughts, I was beginning to wonder precisely that, myself.

*   *   *

I went before the Deferment Board the following week. The Brigadier from the War Department who took the chair was everything one imagined of an established military man. Sharpfaced, shorthaired, resplendent in much-embroidered khaki and displaying an arrogance of bearing, even when seated. In marked contrast, the National Farmer's Union representative was a small chapel-suited man with a profusion of grey hair and a twinkle in his eye — a Welshman, by name, Eifion Pritchard. The third member of the Board was from the Ministry of Agriculture Veterinary Department — a red faced bespectacled Scot who, more often than not, looked over the tops of his glasses rather than through them.

The Brigadier, who had come from London, obviously intended to justify his visit and took a considerable time explaining to me, for I appeared to be the only one listening, how defence strategy for the country was formulated and on what and whom it depended. He developed his theme into the role of our great Nation in an unsettled world and concluded his speech with: 'Mr Lasgarn. Our country always was and always will be a vital force in world peace.' Then, he fixed me with a glare, rather like the chap pointing his finger on the old 'Your Country Needs You' posters, to whom the Brigadier had a sinister familiarity. 'The role is ours!' he continued, releasing me from his glare and raising his eyes to look beyond, as if gazing towards a glorious cinematic sunrise or sunset. 'And we must be worthy of it!'

When he finished, there was a silence, as if space had been left for some recognition of his oratory, such as a small fanfare of trumpets, a round of applause or at least a few 'Hear hears'. But there was nothing, for the Ministry Vet was peering out through the window at a red bricked wall and Mr Pritchard, I suspected, was sleeping with his eyes open.

The Brigadier then asked if my father was in the Army, did I consider myself Military material and was I ever in the Boy Scouts. To all three of which, I answered, 'No'.

The Ministry Vet was then asked for comment. He looked over the tops of his specs and said: 'Remember, there's more to life than calving cows!' I remember thinking what a cynical old fart he was, and wondering whose side he was on. Odd though it was, there was some sense in what he said, but at that stage in my life it was imperceptible.

Then it was Eifion Pritchard's turn. He asked me where I was born and what farming experience I had and, when I mentioned Brynheulog, his face lit up and he banged the table with his fist.

'David Morgan!' he erupted. 'Darw! What a man! I could tell you some tales, Mr Lasgarn. Would you believe that David and I courted the same girl for two years? D'you know what...' The Brigadier coughed and pulled his moustache irritably. 'Another time,' said Eifion Pritchard. 'Another time.'

That was all, and three days later I received a letter giving me deferment, time unspecified, subject to a three weeks' availability.

Eight

Bob Hacker and McBean seemed very pleased that I was now on a more permanent basis in the practice. My salary went up by two pounds a week to fifteen pounds and I gave Brad an extra fifteen bob towards my keep.

One afternoon a few weeks later, things were quiet and I was tidying the boot of my car in the yard at the back of the surgery, when Bob drove in, in his Ford Pilot. All my equipment was strewn about like a gypsy encampment.

'Having a sort out?' he called and came over, hands in pockets, to scrutinise the array. 'That looks as if it's had its day,' he remarked, motioning to the battered medical case which he had given me when I started.

'The drawers are broken as well,' I added. 'I had a cow with a potato jammed in its throat yesterday. But the biggest job was getting my case open!'

Bob smiled. 'Well, we'll have to see what we can do to improve on that,' he said amiably, and walked off down the yard to the surgery.

When I had finally cleaned, sorted and re-arranged the kit, I also went down to the surgery and bumped into Bob, who was coming to see me.

'Got a minute?' he asked, and we went into reception where he leaned upon the sacred counter. 'You never met father, did you, Hugh?' he began. I shook my head. 'Fine vet,' continued Bob. 'Dedicated to his work, and he had such a keen, enquiring mind. Though he was my father, I still don't mind telling you, Hugh, his death was a tragic loss to the profession. Mind, he didn't suffer fools gladly, and if a beast wasn't tied up or ready, or the box hadn't been cleaned and strawed down, he'd play merry hell. But the clients loved and respected him, to a man.' Bob shook his head, obviously still very upset.

'Yes,' I said, 'I was sorry not to be able to meet your father. When they knew, at Glasgow, that he had accepted me, the Dean said that, even though I was only coming for a short while, the experience would be invaluable.' Bob Hacker nodded in agreement.

'Scientific acumen was only part of his nature, for when it came to learning, he was only too ready to share it. We had students from all over the world coming to see practice here and observe his clinical technique. He wanted to pass on all his findings and experience to the oncoming generation of veterinary surgeons, never jealously guarding his discoveries to capture all the credit. But you'll benefit from it, Hugh,' he continued, 'even though it's only indirectly, by seeing the way we tackle things here.' With that, he bent down behind the counter. 'Sadly,' he said, 'the old man won't be here to help you, but at least this will.' And from behind the sacred counter, he raised his father's leather medical bag — the one I'd used on my very first case. 'I'd like you to have this,' said Bob, handing it to me.

'But wouldn't you like it?' I replied, quite taken aback by Bob's offer.

'I've got the one that he bought me when I qualified,' he explained. 'No. You have it, Hugh. I know he would have liked that and I'm sure that if you're stuck, the old man will open the right drawers for you.'

It was like getting my spurs or being capped. I didn't know what to say.

'Go and see if it'll fit in your car,' said Bob and he turned away, pretending to look for something on the top shelf.

So I just said: 'Thank you, I do appreciate it,' and went back out into the yard with G. R. Hacker's leather case gripped firmly in my hand.

* * *

If the spirit of G. R. Hacker, through his medical case, guided me through my first months in practice, there were occasions when I think that even the great man himself would have been stumped.

One evening, a small tousle-headed girl appeared at the surgery, carrying a cardboard box. She placed it carefully upon the floor and out of it took a tortoise.

'When he eats his jaw "clicks",' she announced. 'You listen!' Then, from a packet, she produced a piece of lettuce and, by waving it before her pet's shell, lured its head into view, whence it started to nibble at her offering. Together, we placed our ears close to the munching jaws and, sure enough, a 'clicking' sound could be heard.

Now, the nutritional aspects of the tortoise had not featured very highly in the university curriculum; in fact, I couldn't remember tortoises ever being mentioned at all.

However, once again, from my Abergranog days, I knew that, after hibernation, these curious creatures took a little time to become completely functional and that joints could be stiff and muscles sluggish for a short time. I suggested a mild lubrication of the jaws and demonstrated how it could be done with some liquid paraffin and a dropper. I prepared a small container of the lubricant and told the little girl to bring it back in a few days if the condition hadn't improved.

So far so good. She appeared perfectly satisfied and replaced her tortoise in the box. She was just about to leave, when she paused, then turned to me and said: 'Mother said to ask you if it was a boy or a girl!'

G. R. Hacker, where are you! I thought. Certainly, when it came to sex, I had learnt quite a bit. Cattle I knew about, horses, pigs, sheep, dogs and cats. I knew about the birds and the bees and even humans — but never, despite my Bachelorate in Veterinary Medicine and Surgery, had I learnt how to sex a tortoise.

'Let me see it again,' I requested.

She took it out of the box and I examined it studiously,

turning it over several times, but its undercarriage, to my eye anyway, was completely devoid of any indication. 'Is this the only one you have?' I enquired. She nodded.

'A female,' I said, thinking that of the two, it was the safer choice, a case of hedging my bet. If it was female and laid eggs — fine. And if it did not, or was male, nothing of any consequence would happen anyway.

After surgery, I popped along to the tiny newsagent's shop across the square, bought a cheap paperback on tortoises and read it avidly.

From then on, though the demand for my expertise in that field would be limited, at least I would be ready; but I often wondered how G. R. Hacker would have handled things.

Sex and reproduction, of course, formed an integral part of livestock farming, in order to perpetuate the species that provided both milk and meat.

But, as I found out a few weeks later, this natural event was causing quite a problem for one family who were clients of the practice.

Amy and Elvira Pugh were spinsters in their fifties, both prim and very proper, who lived at Yew Tree Cottage with their father, Abe, a cantankerous, arthritic old man who at one time had been head chauffeur to Mr John Baraby at Great House. Service and respect had been Abe Pugh's maxim and now, in his ninetieth year, he spent his days ordering his daughters about, criticising the progress of the farmers around him and, from his wheelchair seat in the sitting room window, watching Uncle Albert and his ancient harem in the paddock at the front of the cottage.

For interest on retiring, Abe had bought the small flock of sheep, a mixture of Kerry and Halfbred ewes and a Clun ram always referred to as Uncle Albert, although on my occasional visits I had never had the temerity to ask why. But now that he was housebound, his aged pets were tended by his daughters under old Abe's eagle eye.

One Saturday morning, Amy and Elvira presented

themselves at surgery, both weighed down with old-fashioned market baskets full of groceries.

'Could we have a word, Mr Lasgarn?' asked Elvira. 'On a private matter.'

'We've been shopping,' added Amy, rather obviously.

'Won't keep you a minute,' continued Elvira. 'We know how busy you are.'

I ushered the sisters into Bob Hacker's office, as he was off for the day, and invited them to take a seat. They deposited their purchases in the middle of the floor and sat very upright, knees and feet together, on the two available chairs. Then they straightened their coat hems, adjusted their collars and generally preened themselves like two little bantam hens.

'How's your father?' I asked.

At that, they stopped preening and Elvira cleared her throat.

'As difficult as ever,' she replied. 'In fact, that's why we've come. Amy and I don't think we can go through it again!'

'Go through what?' I enquired.

'Lambing!' she said, folding her arms and looking away with an air of disgust. 'They're too old for it. And anyway, it's not fair on us.'

'We were up every night for three weeks last time,' chipped in Amy. 'Father would have us go out every hour. Then, only three had lambs and when one of those died, he went wild and blamed us.'

'How many have you got now?' I asked.

'Only five — and Uncle Albert,' said Elvira. 'And the two lambs.'

'And he won't sell?'

'SELL!' Elvira retorted, sharply. 'We only mentioned that once.'

Amy shook her head and I got the message.

'How about isolating Albert?' I suggested.

'We thought of that, but he wouldn't hear of it. Against "nature" he says and there's no way he'll have that. Even

201

if we tried, he'd know, because he watches them all day from his chair.'

I was about to broach the subject of radical surgical intervention, when Elvira stood up and, turning away from me, faced the wall.

'Amy and I have been talking,' she said, 'and we wondered if Uncle Albert could have the "operation".'

There was a complete silence and Amy bowed her head and studied her boots.

'Nothing too severe,' continued Elvira haltingly, and still with her back to me. 'But I've been reading that there is an operation that will let him ... do what he has to do ... and not give us any lambs.'

'A vasectomy,' I said, thoughtfully.

Elvira turned and Amy looked up, both to stare appealingly into my face.

'YES!' they chorused.

'It's quite possible,' I agreed, averting my eyes from their intense gaze. 'It is being done on rams and the technique is quite straightforward.'

In fact, vasectomised rams were being used experimentally, not just for birth control, but in work to assist the 'synchronisation of oestrus'. This somewhat impersonal scientific term meant bringing all the flock to peak conception at the same time. One idea was to insert 'sheep sponges', which sounded like a Women's Institute speciality, but were actually impregnated tampons that shut down the ovaries and, when removed, allowed them to start up again. A flock impregnated with the 'sponges' should all come into season at the same time after they were removed and, if fertilisation took place, all lamb within a week of each other.

Another method was to introduce a vasectomised ram or 'teaser' into the flock a few weeks before conception was required. The presence of the male stimulated the ewes to become receptive and, once they were all active, the poor 'teaser' was removed and the 'entire' chaps took over.

It all seemed slightly immoral, but that was the way

things were going.

Some of the research work was being done at Glasgow University and, for that reason, I was familiar with the operation; to my mind it seemed the ideal solution.

'The only thing is,' said Elvira who, by then, was seated again, 'Father mustn't know.'

'How can we arrange that?' I asked her. 'You can't bring Albert here, he'll soon notice that.'

'Could you come when Father's in bed?' asked Elvira.

'Any time after ten,' added Amy. 'He wouldn't know then.'

It all sounded a bit clandestine, but I agreed to go the following Thursday night and, after receiving a multitude of thanks, saw the sisters and their shopping baskets on their way.

It was pitch black as I turned into the lane the following Thursday night and I was surprised to find Amy waiting there with a light, for it was a good quarter of a mile from the cottage.

'We thought you'd better leave your car here, just in case Father heard. He's got ears like an elephant,' she said, rubbing her hands nervously.

Together we carried the equipment down the lane and up the paddock to a wooden barn in the far corner. Inside, illuminated by two tilly lamps, stood Elvira clad in a green rubber apron, wellingtons, a mob cap and pink kitchen gloves. Beside her stood three buckets of steaming water and, on a small table, a pile of towels.

I didn't know what Elvira was expecting, but she was certainly well prepared. Uncle Albert was penned behind a gate in the corner and looked completely unconcerned.

'Is there anything else you require, Mr Lasgarn?' asked Elvira importantly, obviously having elected herself as theatre assistant.

'A wheelbarrow,' I replied. 'I saw one down by the pump.'

Elvira looked at me in disbelief. 'A wheelbarrow?' she

repeated.

'Turned up against the wall, it makes an ideal operating chair for this sort of thing,' I explained. 'We sit Uncle Albert in it, tie his hind legs to the handles and, with a rope around his middle, we'll be finished in two shakes.'

The operation went well. With a local anaesthetic, the old fellow didn't feel a thing. After making my incisions into the scrotal wall, I parted out the spermatic cord, removed a section about one and a half inches long and ligated the free ends. Skin sutures, dressings, antibiotic injection and the job was completed.

'Sorry we can't ask you in for a cup of tea,' apologised Amy. 'Father.'

'I understand,' I said. 'Uncle Albert's skin sutures will dissolve in due course, so I shan't need to call again.'

The sisters inundated me with thanks and I bade them goodnight, then made my way down the lane and back to my car.

As I approached, I could discern someone standing beside it, and as I drew nearer discovered it to be PC Bob Packham, leaning on his bicycle.

'Wondered where you were,' he said. 'Knew it was yours. Everything all right?'

I thanked him and assured him that it was.

'Working late,' he commented, in a slightly suspicious tone.

'Been doing a vasectomy on Uncle Albert for Amy and Elvira,' I explained. 'Had to do it at night, so that their father wouldn't know.'

'I see,' said PC Packham, a trifle vaguely.

He didn't say another word after that, just shone his torch for me to put my kit in the boot and moved to one side as I turned the car.

As I drove away, I could see through my mirror that he was still standing in the road, torch in hand, with a bemused look upon his face.

He had given the impression that he understood, but to be quite honest, I didn't think he really had.

The next time I met PC Packham I was again involved with sheep, but the circumstances were very different. Yet it enabled me, in one way, partly to repay a debt that I owed.

Ringing Ledingford were several family farms that ran small dairy herds and raised pigs, hens, fat cattle and sheep and, because of their proximity to the town, found a ready sale for their produce. For the farmers so situated, being close to the built-up area thus had a very real advantage, but there were disadvantages, too. One of these was sheep-worrying by stray dogs.

In fact, it was such a case that brought me one Monday morning to Holyoak Farm, set on the fringe of a council estate to the north of the town. Ivor Barret farmed it and had asked for confirmation that a lamb he had found dead was the victim of such an act; I had been called to conduct a post mortem examination on the unfortunate creature.

I had visited Holyoak twice before to attend to Ivor's cows, so Mrs Barret recognised me when I arrived. A worn, greyhaired woman, she emerged from a door at the side of the house, accompanied by a great issue of steam. Her wrap-around pinafore was wet and her bare arms reddened and soapy from the washing in which she was obviously engaged. Below, she wore large, oversize wellingtons, which suggested that her work was not just confined indoors.

'Oh, Mr Lasgarn,' she called, wringing her arms to shake off the foam. 'Ivor's round the back of the barn looking at the lamb. Constable Packham's there as well.' Mrs Barret pointed to the sturdy, black Raleigh cycle with a black cape folded over the crossbar.

'Worrying business,' she continued. 'Difficult enough to make a decent living without losing them like this. You'll find them all right . . . round by the barn.' With that information delivered, still wringing her arms but now shaking her head as well, she turned and disappeared back into the cloud of steam.

Most of the sheds at Holyoak were black-tarred tin; the barn, a three-bay Dutch type, stood behind the farmhouse, and as I rounded the corner I found Ivor and PC Bob Packham standing by a wheelbarrow in which lay the mauled carcase of a lamb, apparently about two months old. It was a grisly sight, with most of the entrails lying to one side and one hind leg completely missing. Bob Packham had been taking notes on a folding pad and peered over his spectacles at me in an exceedingly serious fashion as I arrived. Amid silence, I stood and studied the remains, then PC Packham flipped back the pages of his pad, coughed and said:

'Mr Lasgarn, sir. Perhaps you would like me to read you the statement of evidence that Ivor, here . . . Mr Barret, has just divulged to me?'

Ivor Barret's thin frame jerked nervously at the realisation that what he had said was now officially a 'statement of evidence'.

'It's true!' he blurted out. 'It's all true!' As if he already anticipated some form of cross examination.

'That would be a good idea,' I replied, a response which the constable had anticipated; but no doubt he would have read it anyway, for he had already adjusted his glasses and assumed the upright posture expected of officers of the Law in the course of reading statements.

Another cough, and he began: 'At seven thirty o'clock this morning, Mr Ivor Barret of Holyoak Farm in the County of Herefordshire . . .' He nodded towards Ivor who appeared to be further startled at this mention of his name in such an official manner. '. . . inspected his flock of Clun-Suffolk crossbred ewes and lambs, totalling fifty ewes and seventy lambs of mixed gender.'

'There's two Shropshire crosses in the ewes,' Ivor corrected.

PC Packham checked his notes, then peered over his glasses at me.

'Significant?' he questioned.

I shook my head.

'Good,' he said, looking back intently at his pad. 'Saves me alterin' it.' Then, following another clearing of his throat, he continued.

The 'statement of evidence' took nearly ten minutes to deliver, the gist of it being that the lamb had been found, dead and mutilated, in the meadow, but the rest of the flock, fortunately, were unharmed. Ivor had suspected dogs, but there were none to be seen. However, just after nine o'clock, he was clearing a drain by the roadside gate, when a black and white collie with bloodstains on its chest came trotting by. Ivor, surprisingly enough, managed to catch the dog and shut it in the barn and, following apprehension of the suspect, had informed the police.

'Pretty open and shut case, Mr Lasgarn,' commented PC Packham, at the conclusion of his epistle. 'You'll certify the carcase?'

'Looks fairly obvious,' I agreed. 'But I'd better open it up and take a closer look to be certain.'

'Good lamb, too,' said Ivor. 'There's too much of this goin' on.'

'How did you manage to catch the dog?' I asked him.

'Called and he come to me. Had a cord round his neck, looked as if he'd been tied up and broke away. Want to see him? He's shut in that shed.' Ivor motioned across the yard and led off towards the small building. 'Look through there, an' you can see him.'

The door was not well fitting, and, through the gap, I saw a foxy little collie lying despondently on some sacks, a long piece of frayed cord trailing from his neck. Sensing my presence, he sat up and gave a sharp bark and, raising his black muzzle, sniffed the air nervously. I studied the roughcoated little dog more closely, for there was something about him that was familiar, but I just couldn't place it.

'Any idea who he belongs to?' I asked Ivor, who was standing at my shoulder.

'Might just 'ave,' he said, thoughtfully. But before I was able to ask him, the answer was provided, as into the yard drove a rusty little red van with the wings loose and flapping.

It juddered to a halt and the engine died, but the body went through a series of convulsions, and puffs of black smoke rose from behind, before it finally became motionless. The driving door creaked open and dropped on its hinges and, with a heave and a grunt, Sam Juggins emerged, red neck-a-chief and all.

Eyeing our trio up and down, his red cheeks rose as a broad grin spread across his face.

'Well, well,' he said. 'Mr Vet Lasgarn and Mr Constable Packham. What 'ave you been up to, Ivor my lad? Caught up with you at last 'ave they?' Chuckling away, he leaned on the bonnet of his dilapidated transport. 'Don' suppose you've seen my dog about? Gone off in the night, the little devil. Bitch in season about somewhere, I wouldn' wonder. Don' suppose you've seen 'im?'

'Thought it might be,' said Ivor Barret. 'Ay, Sam. We got one here in this shed.' With that, he unlatched the door and had only part opened it when a black flash shot through the gap onto the yard.

'Snap!' shouted Sam. 'Sit!'

The collie froze, then sank to the ground, ears pricked, eyes bright, mouth open, its pink tongue jerking with every urgent breath.

'Come!' Sam called, and the dog streaked to his side and sat, looking up at him expectantly. Sam glanced downwards and pulled one of the collie's ear flaps in gentle recogniton.

'Aye. 'E's mine,' he said. 'What's 'e s'pose to have done?'

After an embarrassed silence, PC Packham spoke:

'We have reason to believe, Sam, that this here dog, what you claim to be yours, by name of . . .'

'Snapper,' said Sam.

'By name of Snapper, was h'involved in an incident

which resulted in the death of a good lamb owned by Ivor, here . . . Mr Ivor Barret of Holyoak Farm.'

'Never in a hundred years,' said Sam. 'Not my Snapper.'

'What about the blood on him?' asked Ivor, pointing to Snapper's chest. Sam Juggins bent down and ran his horny fingers through the dog's ruff.

'Blood all right,' he admitted. 'But who's to say it's from your lamb?'

'Come on, Sam,' said Ivor. 'You and I be good neighbours and I'm sorry for your dog. But you knows as well as I do that once a dog takes to killing, there's only one thing to do. Shoot 'im!'

Sam Juggins' countenance had lost all its jollity. He seemed suddenly drained of energy and looked aged and unsteady. Then he turned to me.

'Now then, Mr Lasgarn. You be the vet, what have you got to say?'

The look in Sam's eyes was appealing, but not compromising. 'You be the vet'. I'd heard that before, too. As I looked at him, his red neck-a-chief seemed to do all the talking. It said: 'Remember me? Strip it out. Get 'im to strip it out.'

'I haven't completed my examination, yet,' I said. 'Might have died from something else and been got at afterwards.'

Nobody commented and I knew why. It was because nobody believed it.

However, I went to my car and took out my box with the knives and gloves and other bits and pieces used in the examination of carcases. They followed me in single file back to the wheelbarrow, Snapper coming as well. And watched in silence as I cut the carcase completely apart.

'There 'ain't no liver,' observed Ivor. 'Shows it's a dog.'

'This all you lost?' asked Sam.

Ivor nodded.

'No other sheep even bit?' furthered Sam.

Ivor shook his head.

'Found it early this morning, did you?' Sam continued.

'Just on light,' replied Ivor.

Sam shook his head slowly and turned away. As if just talking to himself, he said: 'That ain't no dog. That's a fox!'

'Definitely been killed by one or the other,' I concluded, after surveying the dismembered carcase. 'Marks on the neck show where it was pulled down and there's no evidence of any disease or other abnormality. Definitely killed.'

'Well it ain't Snapper,' Sam retorted, a trifle aggressively. 'He's too good with sheep for that!'

'He has got a nasty side, though,' PC Packham said sternly. 'When I seen him in the market in your van, he was vicious, Sam. An' Mr Lasgarn will bear me out.'

'He was, Sam,' I admitted.'

'Course 'e is in the van. Course 'e is,' said Sam. 'God bless us, that's where 'e sleeps, an he's only guarding it. But out of there, he's as gentle as they come. How did you catch him, then, Ivor?'

'Just called him, an' he ran to me,' said Ivor.

'There you are, then,' appealed Sam, bending and ruffling Snapper's coat. 'No sheep killer would do that, now would they?'

'Where's the blood from, then?' persisted Ivor.

'Rabbiting.' Sam held up his hand as if that must obviously be the reason, but it failed to convince.

'The circumstantial evidence is very considerable,' commented PC Packham, as if he were the judge summing up.

'Look, Sam,' said Ivor, 'I don't want to get you into court. If you'll put the dog down, I'll stand the loss of the lamb.' Sam shook his head. 'If you don't want to shoot him, I'll do it for you,' added Ivor.

'He never done it.' Sam turned and faced me squarely. 'Dogs work by day and don't just take one lamb. They'll rag the whole flock, tearing and ripping. Then they'll run off, hardly ever eat anything. Leave alone take a leg away. Can't you do anything, Mr Lasgarn? I don't want to shoot this little dog.'

And Snapper pushed tight against Sam's baggy

trousers, as if he understood all that was being said.

It was Mrs Barret, hanging out her washing at the back of the house, who gave me the idea. As the sheets and shirts blew gaily in the wind I was reminded of a visit I had made with C. J. Pink to a farm where a collie, not unlike Snapper, was thought to have swallowed poison. And that was a Monday, too.

'Has your wife got any washing soda, Ivor?' I asked.

The three men looked at me as if I had taken leave of my senses; even Snapper seemed to raise his foxy head in amazement.

'Washing soda?' questioned Ivor.

'Yes,' I said. 'A piece about as big as my thumbnail, that's all.'

Ivor crossed to the house and shortly returned, followed by Mrs Barret. She looked equally incredulous as she held out a box.

'Is this what you want?' she asked. 'It's proper washing soda.'

I selected a small lump and turned to Sam.

'I want you to give this to your dog. Open his mouth and pop it down.'

Sam didn't question my motive. He took the washing soda, sniffed it, then, bending down, opened Snapper's jaws and pushed it far to the back of the collie's throat. The dog wriggled, but Sam held his mouth firmly closed until a gulp signalled that the soda had been swallowed.

'What now?' asked Sam.

I didn't answer, for I knew that, if it worked, as it had when C. J. Pink had used it, the results would soon be obvious.

We stood around peering down at Sam's dog, which he was still holding by the cord.

'Let him go, Sam,' I advised. As Sam released the cord, Snapper got up and circled twice in front of us. Then he whined uneasily and started to heave. Still heaving he ran a few yards, then stopped and was violently sick.

It wasn't a pretty sight by any means, and poor Snapper

211

went through extreme discomfort for several minutes. But it proved a point. Sam had been right, for there, for all to see, were the remains of a partly digested rabbit.

PC Packham surveyed the evidence, then wrinkled up his nose.

'We'll continue with our enquiries, Ivor,' he said, folding up his notepad. 'But I think we can release the suspect, pending further h'investigation.'

'Aye,' said Ivor, 'that's proof enough. Sorry about it, Sam, but what was I to think?'

'Don' worry about it,' he replied, as he comforted Snapper who was now lying down, completely exhausted. 'Thanks, Mr Lasgarn.'

'Not at all, Sam.' I looked him straight in the eye. 'I was glad I could help you.'

'One good turn . . .' he said.

I nodded 'You're right,' I agreed, then added, 'Good job it was Monday.'

But he didn't get the point.

*   *   *

Through my veterinary work I was meeting more and more folk every day, discovering more characters and making more friends.

But I was losing some as well. Brad's old cat, Percy, was killed outside the digs one evening, by a motorcyclist. It was about three weeks after I had removed the wire frame from his jaw which had healed remarkably well, much to Brad's pleasure. But that must have been Percy's ninth life and, when the motorbike came along, his credit had run out. Charlie left, too. He went to Chester to open another butcher's shop, and I missed his happy-go-lucky company tremendously.

But the biggest change in my life was Diana.

The Spring of that year for me was definitely a time of discovery. I discovered the art of veterinary medicine, the beauty of the countryside and a degree of happiness and

enthusiasm for life I had never thought possible.
And I discovered I was in love.

Nine

As the weeks rolled by I came to realise that veterinary work, like the farming to which it was so closely allied, was more a way of life than just a job. I had realised that time was of little consequence to my patients and that the cow that had difficulty in calving at two in the morning, or the horse that decided to develop colic at Sunday lunchtime, did it without any thoughts of conforming to a nine-to-five pattern, or even to a six-day week.

But as the seasons marked the major changes in rural life in a gradual manner, so were there certain more specific landmarks in the country calendar by which time was measured.

Ledingford Agricultural and Horse Show was one of them. Snippits of conversation could often be heard that admirably demonstrated this feature, such as:

'When did you dip yer sheep?' — 'Oh, two weeks afore the Show.' Or, 'Now tell me, Beth, when did they get married?' — 'About a month after the Show.' Or, 'I had mumps last year, just on Show time!' Ledingford Show was, indeed, a supremely important occasion, giving relief from work and a day out for honest competition, paying bills, meeting friends, drinking cider and having fun.

The Hacker practice were Honorary Veterinary Surgeons to the Society and attended on the day; but when the day came round, Bob Hacker was taking his summer break and McBean suggested that, once the urgent calls had been cleared, I should represent the practice.

I had previously arranged to pick up Diana from work at

eleven o'clock and arrived just outside the offices of Seamer's dead on time. It was, however, a quarter of an hour before she burst through the main door looking delightfully flustered. She wore a white dress with a full skirt that had differently coloured flowers printed on it and was gathered at the waist by a narrow rope belt. The neckline was wide but not low, allowing her long blonde hair to cover bare, sun-browned shoulders.

I cast a veterinary eye over her for, up until meeting Diana, I had never taken the opposite sex very seriously and regarded them mainly as a necessary attachment only if one went to a dance. In Abergranog there had been girls, but they were different in that they had different playgrounds, different games, different lavatories, and we boys were rather scornful of their company, having far more important things on our minds. At university I had met several girls, but on a student allowance in those days it was difficult to create much of an impression. So I settled for Rugby and snooker and bawdy songs in the Student Union bar.

But as this vision came towards the car, smiling happily, I discarded my veterinary eye without delay, accepting that, while it was sometimes possible to credit animals with human attributes, a beautiful girl could never be anything but a beautiful girl — and in Diana's case, the effect on a young country vet was devastating!

If that wasn't enough, when she got in, the little Ford became filled with such an exotic perfume that it was a wonder its wheels didn't fall off, for my legs certainly felt detached. I sat back, closed my eyes and took a deep breath.

'Mmm! That must be the most beautiful smell in the world,' I said, inhaling deeply for the second time.

'Well, you should know,' replied Diana, laughingly. 'All vets are experts on smells.'

'Not like that,' I admitted. 'No, ma'am! Not like that.'

'Carven, "Ma Griffe".' Diana held out her arm, turned it upwards and slowly passed it beneath my nose.

215

'There should be a Home Office licence on stuff like that,' I said, recovering slightly.

'Don't you like it?' she asked, sniffing the back of her hand to reassure herself.

'You should have a red ribbon in your hair whenever you wear it,' I told her and, taking another lungful, pulled away from the kerb.

Ledingford Show was held in the grounds of Granstone Castle, on parkland that sloped gently down to the river. The estate was the home of Lord Pendleford and a glorious setting for one of the best one-day displays of livestock and agricultural produce in the Borders. For most of the year, the rolling pastures, overlooked by Granstone, a fine castellated mansion, were populated solely by ancient oaks and grazing cattle. But at Show Time, like magic mushrooms, tents and marquees sprouted overnight, and multicoloured banners and high-flying flags fluttered merrily overhead. It became an encampment full of hustling, bustling, happy country folk and superbly bred animals, focusing the attention of the whole county, and further afield if anyone was prepared to note, on all that was good in agriculture.

There was a queue of cars at the entrance which had been divided into two avenues, separated by rope, each guarded by stewards with armbands and large poacher's bags in which they were depositing the money. When our turn came, a rather toffee-nosed chap in tweeds and a deerstalker pushed his hand through the window and said, haughtily: 'One pound!'

What followed gave me immense pleasure, especially as Diana was with me, for out of my pocket I took the badge which Bob Hacker had left for whichever of us attended the Show.

'Veterinary Surgeon,' I replied, equally haughtily.

'Veterinary Surgeon,' he repeated, looking at me suspiciously. Then another steward leaned over his shoulder, eyed the badge and said: 'Vet. Official cars on the left.' At which instruction, I revved up the little Ford as grandly as I was able and drove off to the left.

'My,' said Diana impishly, 'it's the first time I've been to the Show with an Official.'

'So who have you been with before?' I asked, as I pulled into line.

'Never you mind,' she said, laughing. 'But it wasn't with an Official!'

From the privileged position of the Official Car Park it was only a short distance to the showground. I bought a programme and spotted amongst the list of names: Hon. Veterinary Surgeon: R. A. Hacker MRCVS.

'There's Bob's name,' I said, underlining it with my finger.

'Should be yours,' commented Diana.

'Might be, one day,' I replied.

'At Ledingford?' She stopped and looked at me wistfully, and I knew it wasn't just a simple question.

'If it was, would you still come with me?' I asked.

Her eyes searched my face eagerly, as if trying to give me an answer for which her lips weren't ready. Then she sidetracked and said: 'If you were an Official, how could I refuse?' Then she took hold of my hand, adding, 'Come on, Mr Vet. Show me the Show!'

As we approached the main ring, the ladies' hunter side-saddle class was entering. Diana stood enthralled by the effortless grace of the riders and the fluent, freeflowing action of their mounts. To me, they appeared as latter day Godivas, darkclad and veiled, aloof, yet courting attention with intriguing sensuality. I was privately contemplating the captivating scene when Diana interrupted my train of thought.

'Hugh!' she cried. 'Can't you hear!'

I broke my reverie, just in time to catch the last words of the loudspeaker announcement.

'. . . urgently to the goats!'

'They want a veterinary surgeon at the goats,' she

explained excitedly. 'Come on, quickly!'

'My case is in the car,' I protested, as she dragged me away from the ring. 'Anyway, where are the goats?'

'Goats is by the sheep,' said a fat man standing next to us. 'Same as always.'

I thanked him for the information which was of little help, as I didn't know where the sheep were, either. However, on the way to collect my case, I passed a sign post with numerous fingers pointing in all directions, and amongst 'Main Ring,' 'Toilets', 'Cattle', 'Horses', 'Pigs' and 'Dog Show', I spied 'Sheep'. With Diana in close attendance, I set off hastily in the direction indicated.

Breathless and uncomfortably warm, we came across the goat tent next to the sheep lines, at the far end of the showground. Because of the hot weather, the flaps of the tent had been rolled up to improve ventilation, revealing a maze of hurdles that sectioned the interior into pens. Each one contained all the bric-a-brac of goatkeeping, with bales of hay, bags of feed, milking buckets, boxes, brushes, halters and, of course, goats. There were drab, mouse-coloured Toggenburgs with swinging tassels; tall, lop-eared Nubians straight out of the Book of Moses; snow-white Saanens and jet black Alpines. Some were busily chewing on bunches of hazel twigs tied to their hurdles, while others looked about with an air of complete disdain, as if it was all a bit beneath them.

A fussy, bowler-hatted little man in a slightly oversize, navy-blue pin-striped suit, came forward, clutching an untidy sheaf of papers.

'Vet?' he enquired anxiously. 'Thank goodness.'

'Hugh Lasgarn.' I held out my hand. 'Where's the emergency?'

'Mr Bevan. Steward of the Goats,' he responded, briefly touching my palm, 'and it's not an emergency. Not yet, anyway,' he blew out his cheeks nervously. 'But it soon could be. It soon could be.'

Noticing Diana, he smiled weakly and touched the rim of his bowler. Then taking me by the elbow, he looked around furtively, like a spy about to pass secret information, and said: 'There's a fellow here with two sets of tack!'

I blinked, so he repeated it. 'Two sets of tack!' This time more slowly and deliberately.

He studied my face eagerly, then assuming, in part correctly, that I hadn't yet got the message, he took hold of my arm and pulled me a few paces further away from Diana. Then, stretching on tip-toe, he came close to my right ear and whispered hoarsely:

''E's got a willy and a wonker!'

I fought hard to suppress my reactions and turned away to look at Diana, who was obviously puzzled by the whole affair.

'A willy and a wonker,' he repeated, this time more loudly. 'You come and see. See for yourself!' And still holding my arm, he propelled me into the tent, steering me through the pens until we arrived at a section where a small, biscuit-coloured goat was busily tucking into a forest of twigs.

Mr Bevan, Steward of the Goats, put down his papers, took off his bowler hat and laid it on top. Then, after looking about nervously once again, he knelt down behind the goat, who seemed completely indifferent to his presence, and thrust his hand between its back legs.

Looking up, he said: 'If you feel under here — there's a willy.' Then, with the other hand, he raised the stumpy tail. 'And if you look under there — there's a wonker! See!'

I took a step forward and a closer look to confirm the remnants of a female orifice, and when Mr Bevan got out of the way, I felt the male appendage beneath the goat's belly.

'Hermaphrodite!' I announced.

Mr Bevan replaced his bowler and shuffled the papers into an even more untidy bundle.

'You knows it an' I knows it, Mr Lasgarn. But the owner don't! Now, I can't enter that goat because, well . . .' He shrugged his shoulders. 'There ain't no call for a Class like that, you see.'

'Should be no problem,' I assured him. 'It's a pretty obvious case.'

'Will you explain it to the owner?' he pleaded. 'You'd know how to put it better than me.'

'Certainly,' I agreed. 'Who is it?'

'She's over there.' He pointed to a tall, rather flamboyantly dressed female, standing with her back towards us. 'Lady Octavia Grimes,' he explained. 'Lord Pendleford's sister!'

I felt the clammy hand of fate settling upon me and looked around accusingly at Mr Bevan.

'Sorry!' he said. 'But I did mention it could be an emergency.'

'Not a diplomatic emergency, though,' I added. But, whatever, there was nothing for it, Her Ladyship would have to be told and I was the victim. Clutching my case, I moved forward, somewhat rigidly, to confront the aristocracy, not having a clue as to how I should broach such a delicate subject.

As I drew near, she turned, and for the first time I saw her, full frontal.

To say she had a strong face was probably the kindest way of putting it. Certainly, it was a large face, accommodating dark eyebrows, deepset eyes and a prominent nose. Her make-up was pale and powdery, contrasting violently with bright red lipstick. A wide-brimmed straw hat attempted to obscure her countenance with flattering shadow, but was fighting a losing battle, and as I approached she seemed to lurch sideways, like a listing windjammer. But, by plunging the point of her unopened parasol deftly into the turf, she arrested her sway in the nick of time.

'Lady Octavia?' I spoke as firmly as I could.

She nodded condescendingly, and a small cloud of powder drifted onto her shoulders.

'Hugh Lasgarn, veterinary surgeon. I've just had a look at your goat.'

She raised a lorgnette that had been dangling on a black cord at her side and scrutinized me closely. Then, having satisfied herself that I merited her attention, but still peering through her glasses, she drew herself up to her full height, which was at least three inches taller than myself, and boomed:

'So you've seen Bertie. What do you think of him?'

I put my case down, cleared my throat and began:

'Bertie's got a bit of a problem.'

'A problem!' she echoed.

'Well, he's a shade abnormal.'

'Abnormal!' she boomed, with such volume that everyone in the vicinity froze. 'Tell me more!' she continued. 'Tell me more!' And with that, everyone nearby instantly unfroze and gathered round.

'By a quirk of nature,' I explained cautiously, 'Bertie has developed hermaphroditic tendencies. He has vestiges of female reproductive organs as well as being equipped with normal male genitalia.' I felt I was making little impression as she stood before me like Boadicea, eyeing me through the glasses and not saying a word. 'It's usually a hormonal imbalance due to circulation of oestrogens in excess of normal, and quite often . . .' But I got no further, for she stirred, raised her hand and, dropping the lorgnette to her side, roared in a stentorian tone that filled the tent:

'You're telling me that Bertie's a bloody will-jill!'

The silence was deafening, broken only by a low moan that came from behind me, which I assumed was Mr Bevan, Steward of the Goats, breathing his last.

Lady Octavia clasped her heavily jewelled hands in front of her and raised her eyes to the tent roof.

I was racking my brains for something to say when she suddenly dropped her hands, threw back her head and burst into a gale of laughter.

The effect of this unpredicted reaction was highly contagious, and the onlookers all fell about with uncontrolled mirth, which I suspected was more through relief than humour.

'Mr Lasgarn,' Lady Octavia exclaimed, tears running down her face, 'you've made my day. Just wait until I tell my brother.'

Mr Bevan, now recovered, came up to us and started to explain why he couldn't enter Bertie for judging, but her Ladyship ignored him and turned again to me.

'You're new, Mr Lasgarn. I assume you are helping young Mr Hacker, now that his dear father is dead. Well, you really have bucked me up, you know. Every Show night my brother gives a dinner party — stuffy old affair usually, awfully boring. But tonight I shall set the conversation alight when I tell them all about Bertie. You obviously haven't been to Granstone, yet. But if you do come to see the animals, call on me, my apartment is in the west wing. I'll show you the rest of my family, I breed Maltese, you know.'

'How many have you?' I enquired.

'Fifty-six,' she said. 'Do call.'

And with that, she swept away between the hurdles, obviously intent on consoling poor Bertie.

Over lunch, I explained the commotion to Diana who had watched the whole episode from a safe distance.

'Sounds as if you made quite a hit there,' she observed. 'Come out with you for a day and already I've got competition.'

'Not really my type,' I assured her. 'Come on, let's go and see the cattle.'

The cattle lines were in an area shaded by oaks on the south side of the showground. There were graceful Ayrshires, solid Shorthorns and widebodied Friesians, but by far the largest entry were the Herefords.

They inhabited what seemed like an endless avenue of stalls, stretching as far as one could see. Magnificent, deep red-coated bulls, the older ones standing patiently while their coats were brushed and tails combed, the younger, more inexperienced ones frisky and keen to get on the move, charged with all the excitement of the occasion. Further down, placid, dreamy-eyed, white-faced cows looked on tolerantly as their calves, like kids out of school, leaped and bawled, tugged on their ropes or eyed the on-lookers mischievously.

As in the goat section, much space was taken up with all the paraphernalia of showing. Great wooden travelling boxes proclaimed the owner's name or herd title in bold letters painted on the lids: 'Merryhill Herefords', 'The Eaton Herd', and other descriptive information that conjured up rich pastoral scenes of fertile, grazing herds. When a lid was opened it revealed a chest full of secrets, guarded jealously by animal-wise stockmen, with salves and ointments, potions and lotions, each one to put some special finishing touch to the final presentation. There were curry combs and brushes, snow-white cotton halters and leather head collars adorned with eyebright brass-ware. And on the inside of the lid, fluttering in the breeze, were the rosettes — red, white, blue and tricolour — in row upon gaudy row, the trophies of past success. And well earned, too, for the art of cattle showmanship was a country talent that took years of experience to perfect; many were the tricks of the trade, not only in preparation but in presentation, when a hardly perceptible movement of a leading rope, a quiet word or nearly inaudible low whistle (which passed unnoticed by the onlooker), could make all the difference between a bull standing up proudly or missing the opportunity to catch the judge's eagle eye.

There was a large crowd ranged around the judging ring, where a group of some twenty maiden Hereford heifers were parading.

'Just like a beauty competition,' said Diana, rising up on her toes to see them.

'Well, they are the girls of the family,' I agreed. 'Go on. Pick the winner.'

A few people moved away in front of us, and we were able to get to the rope that separated the spectators from the action.

'They all seem the same to me,' Diana remarked, shaking her head. 'What is the judge looking for?'

'Poise, balance, a good figure,' I replied. 'Just like bathing beauties.'

The judge, a portly gentleman in a dark suit and bowler, had his back to us. He had drawn out five heifers to stand in line before him, obviously his final selection, and was about to decide upon the order. Moving up and down the line, he prodded rumps, probed flanks and moved one animal up a place, then put one down. Eventually, satisfied with his selection, he tapped the winner on the back with a silver-topped cane — and when he turned round I could see it was none other than Paxton of Donhill.

As the heifers left the ring, he surveyed the crowd, and when his eyes fell upon me, he bounced his cane several times on the ground and then came across.

'Well, Lasgarn,' he barked, glaring at me as if I had criticised his judgement. 'Agree with that?'

'You're the judge, Mr Paxton,' I replied diplomatically.

'Correct!' he boomed. 'There's only one person in this ring I've got to please. That's myself!'

Then his eye strayed to Diana and, as if by magic, his frosty glare melted into a benevolent smile, the like of which I would never have imagined him capable.

'Mr . . .' I nearly got it wrong, but corrected myself in the nick of time. 'Diana. This is Mr Paxton of Donhill. Mr Paxton — Diana . . .'

The old tyrant held the brim of his immaculate bowler and raised it elegantly.

'My pleasure, young lady,' he beamed. 'My pleasure.'

Diana responded with a delectable smile, then Paxton again rounded on me.

'Don't know what you've done to deserve company like this, Lasgarn — you're a very fortunate fellow, d'y hear!' He caught sight of the next Class entering the ring. 'Excuse me, but I must get back to work,' he said softly to Diana.

He was on the point of leaving when, once again, he fixed me with his steely glare.

'Oh, yes,' he said, 'I want you to cut the corns out of Warrior. I want it done soon. Ring me tomorrow.' Then he stalked back to the judging.

It was like a knife in the back. 'Cut the corns out of Warrior — soon.' For the second time in hours I felt in a state of shock; the first had been having to break the truth to Lady Octavia, which had fortunately gone all right. But now Warrior, this was a different affair. My mind flashed back to McBean's relief when I told him Paxton didn't consider my suggestion. What did he say? 'If that Warrior should snuff it while you're cutting away at his corns . . . it's "Boom! Boom! Goodbye Hugh"!' And with Bob Hacker away — oh, my God, this was trouble.

'What a nice man,' said Diana, running her fingers through her hair. 'D'you know, I think he liked me. You can have your old Lady Octavia Grimes.'

'Of the two, I would much prefer her at this minute,' I said. 'I just wish we hadn't met him this afternoon.'

'Why on earth not?' asked Diana.

I explained about my precipitous advice on Warrior's condition when I had visited Donhill some months previously, and the responsibility that I had unwittingly let myself in for.

'Why did I open my big mouth?' I droned. 'A mad flight of fancy, and now the bird is coming home to roost.'

'Surely it can't be that dangerous,' comforted Diana. 'And it can't be that difficult. You should see my grandmother, she's terrific at it. Does all her old friends quite regularly.'

'Oh, Diana,' I said, chuckling, 'I'm sure she does, but her "old friends" don't weigh over a ton, like mine does.'

I tried to put the prospect of the operation to the back of my mind during the rest of the afternoon as we enjoyed all the Show had to offer.

I attended the victims of a fight at the Dog Show, where two Jack Russells had a difference of opinion which resulted in one losing a chunk from his right ear. The owner enquired, quite innocently, if I could stitch it back on, which I explained was not possible. Then some wag standing nearby suggested I cut a piece out of the other ear to match, and that nearly started another fight.

About five o'clock, I was called to the horse boxes, where a hunter had been cut at the back of a hind fetlock.

'Don't think you can do much,' the chap in charge informed me. 'But I just want you to check that it hasn't damaged the tendon.'

It was a horizontal wound, but not gaping and quite clean. Fortunately it was only the skin that was broken and none of the underlying tissues were affected. I cleansed and disinfected the area and packed it with sulphonamide powder.

'What's the tetanus status?' I asked.

'He's been vaccinated recently, so he should be all right,' came the reply.

'How did it happen?' Diana enquired.

'That mule over there,' said the groom aggressively, pointing to a classy looking bay mare tied beneath a tree. 'It isn't fair on unsuspecting folks. With a kick like that, she ought to be wearing a red ribbon!'

'Red ribbon!' Diana flashed an indignant glance in my direction. 'Why a red ribbon?'

'Approach with caution, miss,' explained the groom. 'That is, unless you wants yer head kicked off!'

My vision rounded upon me, hands on hips.

'Carven "Ma Griffe",' I said defensively.

'No, his name's Sailor,' said the groom.

'You wait till I get you alone,' said Diana, and even Sailor looked round enviously, while the groom made a 'clicking' sound with his mouth and gave me a broad wink.

And wishing both man and horse 'Goodbye', I beat a hasty retreat to the car.

But Diana's pique was shortlived and we spent the evening at a quaint riverside pub called The Sallies, to end a most eventful day. As I lay in bed that night, I thought to myself what wonderful company she had been and how I was fully in agreement with old Paxton that I was a most fortunate fellow.

But when I closed my eyes all I could see was Warrior, hobbling up and down before me, complaining bitterly about his wretched corns.

As I drove to the surgery the following morning, I deliberated how I might avoid operating upon the great bull; perhaps Paxton might change his mind. But my chances of reprieve diminished when, on arrival, Miss Billings informed me that he had already rung twice, in order to speak to me.

When I got through, Paxton was in his usual, arrogant form.

'I want it done tomorrow, Lasgarn,' he roared.

'But Mr Hacker is away and I haven't been able to speak to Mr McBean,' I explained — which was quite true as McBean had already taken two early calls.

'What in hell's name has that got to do with it!' he almost screamed. 'I asked you! Not anybody else!'

'Yes, but — it's a big job and there are risks.'

My reply was greeted with a hollow silence, as if the line had gone dead, but I surmised from previous experience, that it was but the lull before a very violent storm. Yet, when he did respond, Paxton's voice was uncannily controlled.

'Now look, young fellow,' he began, in a threateningly sinister tone. 'Don't you talk to me of risks.' Then his voice rose gradually in a crescendo. 'Don't you talk to me of bloody risks. I know about risks — and you are a professional and professionals have to take risks. You've trained, God knows how many years, at that university . . .'

'Five,' I interjected, amazed that I was able to get a word in, in spite of his tirade. But Paxton was only drawing breath, for immediately he bore on:

'You're supposed to know — otherwise I'd do the bloody job myself, d'y hear! Now I want you here tomorrow morning at ten-thirty — and no buts!' I heard him draw breath again. 'Any instructions?' he asked finally.

That was an invitation to be very rude if I had had the courage, but that would probably have inflamed the situation irreparably.

'Starve him,' I said, quite involuntarily, as if my body had accepted the commitment even if my mind had not.

'Any water?' he asked.

'Not after five o'clock,' I advised.

'Right, Lasgarn. Tomorrow!' And with that, he slammed down the phone.

For a few minutes, I sat quite still, just meditating.

'You all right, Mr Lasgarn?' asked Miss Billings.

'Yes, thanks, just fine,' I lied. 'Just fine.'

McBean's face was a picture when I told him what had been arranged.

'Mother Mary and all the Saints be blessed,' he said, and gave a low whistle.

'Sorry Mac,' I apologised. 'But somehow I feel I got pushed into it.'

'Now that's nothing to be ashamed of,' he said, rubbing his chin thoughtfully. 'That divil would push his grandmother's tits through a mangle, just for the laugh!' He looked straight at me, and I had to smile — there was no doubt about it, McBean could certainly put things in perspective, regardless of the intensity of the problem. 'You told him the risks?' I gave a confirmatory nod. 'It'll have to be done, an' that's for sure,' he affirmed, slapping his thigh. 'So, Hugh, me laddo. Let's get it organised.'

'You'll help me?' I asked.

'Sure an' I will,' he replied. 'Now, Bob has anaesthetised several bulls with chloral and mag sulph. It's as safe as you'll get and fairly gentle. Bit of a swine if it gets outside the vein.'

'Like what?' I enquired.

'Irritant. Causes a slough and half the neck drops off!'

228

'Oh, Mac,' I said, 'what did I let us in for? You must think I'm the perfect idiot.'

Mac scrutinized me closely, then shook his head and said with a grin, 'No I don't, Hugh. None of us is perfect!'

For an hour we discussed the operation step by step. How much anaesthetic, how long it would last. How to prevent inhalation of rumenal contents and how to prevent bloat. What to do in case of haemorrhage, how deep to incise, and care during the recovery stage. At the end, I felt more confident and, knowing I would have McBean's assistance, I was reassured and even mildly looking forward to the challenge.

I prepared all the equipment before leaving surgery that night and read through my lecture notes several times before I turned in.

Come what might, I was as ready as I could be.

*   *   *

I had started doing morning surgeries, and the following day, before I was able to get off to Donhill, I had to deal with a dog that had a sore paw and one with an ulcerated eye, and I had to castrate a cat. At five past nine, Miss Billings, who had taken well to my innovation, shepherded in the last client.

'Billy Bent and his budgerigar,' she announced, sounding as if it was a Music Hall act. But it was no spectacle of gaiety and joy that met my eyes as Billy, cap in hand, struggled into the exotic plant consulting room carrying a cage covered with a piece of drab curtain material.

On the contrary, it was a sad little combination, for Billy was about eight years old, pale and red eyed as if he had been crying. His pullover was typical of the joke about holes being held together with wool and his short trousers, well above his nobbly, scabby knees, were extensively patched. From the top of his basin-cut hairstyle to his oversize, uncomfortable looking boots, he was barely more than three foot six and hardly high enough to put his cage on the table. I took it from him and removed the cover.

Sitting forlornly at the edge of the perch and leaning against the wire, was a blue budgerigar whose physical appearance matched its tiny owner's pathetic state. The bird's plumage was drab and lack-lustre, its eyes half closed as if dozing, but occasionally, it jerked itself awake, only just in time to avoid toppling from its perch.

'It's his stomach,' said Billy. 'It's all swollen up. My sister said I fed him too much, but I never,' the little boy rubbed his eyes and looked away.

Without even handling it, I could see the protrusion at its front, which was no doubt the cause of the imbalance.

'How long has he been like this?' I asked.

'Nearly a week,' said Billy, sniffing hard. 'Will he die?'

It was a simple question, asked so openly and expectantly and without any intention of putting responsibility upon me. And yet it had. It was as bad as Paxton, yet so different.

How did I know whether it would die or live? Who did he think I was? I'm a professional, I told myself grimly — I'm supposed to know — supposed to accept responsibility.

So why didn't I say: 'I don't know'? As I should have with Paxton. Then, I wouldn't have been sweating on the top line about Warrior. Be cautious; hedge; don't commit yourself. But how on earth could I help it?

'What do you call him, Billy?' I asked, looking down at the little chap.

'Peter,' he said, his voice quivering.

'He won't die, Billy,' I said confidently. 'Not if I can help it.'

I managed to catch the frail creature without much effort and, holding it carefully, wings pinioned, in the palm of my hand, I turned it onto its back.

Gently I probed the swelling, which was generally soft and pliable. It was obviously an impaction of the crop.

When I questioned Billy about the feeding, he replied bluntly, 'Seed and greens.'

But there was no grit in the cage and I explained to the lad how budgies needed the sharp insoluble mixture to aid digestion.

'Ask your Dad to get you some,' I told him. 'It's quite cheap.'

'Me Dad's dead,' he replied, stony-faced.

'I'm sorry to hear that, Billy,' I apologised. 'Your Mam, then.'

'Mam's in the General,' he informed me matter-of-factly. 'She's got a growth.' He put his hands in his trouser pockets and kicked an imaginary football across the surgery floor. I put my hand on his shoulder.

'Look, Billy,' I said. 'You come back tonight and I'll have some for you. In the meantime, we'll give Peter a tiny dose of liquid paraffin to ease his stomach.'

'He won't die, will he?' he asked again.

I shook my head. 'Bring him back tonight,' I said. 'There's a good lad.'

As Billy left, McBean came through to see how I was getting on.

'There's a call at Connelly's, I'll go round that way and see to it, then I'll come over to Donhill. You take the gear and get things set up and I'll join you as soon as I can. I expect Paxton will be champing at the bit, but don't let him rattle you. Okay?'

'Okay,' I agreed. 'I'll check the instruments and see you there.'

McBean was dead right, for even though I was a quarter of an hour early, the old man was impatient for action and bore down upon me before I could even get out of the car.

'Mr McBean will be along shortly, to give a hand,' I informed him, but it was more to give myself confidence than to appease Paxton.

'Two vets!' he exclaimed, irritably. 'Huh!'

I was about to explain how difficult the anaesthesia could be with a great bull like Warrior, but decided against it. I was committed to the operation and it was no good arguing the toss with him, in his evidently truculent mood.

'I've had the big yard strawed down,' he announced, rattling his cane on the concrete. 'It's partly covered, so there's no draughts and nothing sharp to cause any problems. There's four men, plenty of rope and gallons of hot water. Anything else?'

Fair play to the man, he was organised, despite his manner.

'Some straw bales to put the instruments on — and then I'd like to give Warrior a checkover before we start,' I replied.

'That bull's as fit as a fiddle,' retorted Paxton. 'Apart from his back legs. But this operation puts them right, so I'm told,' he continued. 'Harper of Kesley in Warwickshire had his bull done last month and it's walking perfectly. I want mine done the same!'

By the time I had examined Warrior it was eleven o'clock, and still no sign of McBean. The bull was, indeed, as fit as a fiddle, though had I found some problem that would have genuinely prevented me carrying out the task, I had to admit, I would not have been unduly displeased. But the heartbeat was strong, the lungs clear and the temperature normal.

'How long will it take?' Paxton asked, as I folded up my stethoscope.

I wasn't really sure, but said 'half an hour', in as positive a manner as I could muster.

By eleven fifteen I was ready, with everything laid out, the chloral warmed up and my hands sweating.

'Where's McBean?' roared Paxton.

'On his way, I hope,' I affirmed, rearranging the order of the instruments for the fourth time.

'I can't have men hanging about like this,' he bellowed, banging his cane on the gatepost. At that moment, a greyhaired woman came across the yard holding a piece of paper. 'A message for Mr Lasgarn,' she said, nervously, 'from the surgery.'

I didn't have to read it — I knew: McBean wasn't coming. When I looked at the note it confirmed my fears. He had been held up and wouldn't be with me for an hour, at least. I would have to tackle it alone.

Paxton was eyeing me closely and I knew that if I asked for a delay, there would be fireworks. So I crumpled up the note, swallowed deeply and said:

'McBean will be late — we'll make a start.'

Anticipation of a demanding occasion is the most harrowing part of the ordeal. I'd heard of famous actors and opera stars, who appeared so confident and professional on stage, suffering similar agonies. Even the greatest had 'butterflies' and some even became physically ill. But once the performance commenced, such was the involvement that there was no time for fear or thought of failure — and the moment I gave myself the signal, miraculously my nervousness vanished.

Warrior was a brick. It took me two stabs to get properly into his jugular which was up like a drainpipe, and yet he never budged. I had Mason and one other man at the head and one man either side of his body, to steady him if possible. As the chloral slowly narcotised the great hulk, Warrior closed his eyes and, in just over a minute, he sank gently to his knees, then lowered his powerful hindquarters and finally lay on his side in perfect position.

I made sure that his air passages were clear and raised his head by packing wedges of straw beneath. Then, with ropes on his hind legs, I dragged them into a position where I could infiltrate the corns with local anaesthetic. When they were adequately frozen and Warrior snoring contentedly, I tied a rope tourniquet around his ankle, disinfected the site and made ready for the incision.

'Corns' are exuberant growths of tissue or 'proud flesh' which can recur if not completely excised. 'Make the cut bold and deep,' my notes had said, and so I did. The cavity left between the clees seemed massive, but the haemorrhage was not excessive and, certainly, there was no evidence of any 'corn' tissue remaining.

I packed it tight with sulphonamide and strapped it firmly with a heavy bandage and tape. Throughout the whole procedure, I had kept a watchful eye on Warrior's chest, always thankful to see it heaving gently up and down.

Then I set to and worked on the other foot, which went equally well. My concentration had made me unaware of time, but as I gave the tape on the final dressing a last twist, Paxton, who had been standing but a yard away throughout the whole proceedings, said: 'Just over half an hour.'

It was then that I became aware of myself again, but this time I felt a degree of euphoria, as I thought with relief: So far — so good.

We sat Warrior upon his brisket and propped him up with bales, then I gave him a large dose of crystalline penicillin directly into his muscle.

'He should be up within an hour,' I commented, feeling far more confident about things.

'Feeding?' interrupted Paxton.

'Just a little hay, later on,' I suggested.

'Tell Mason,' said Paxton gruffly. 'You'll check him tomorrow?'

'Yes,' I affirmed. Then, without a word of thanks or criticism, the old man grunted, turned on his heels and, flourishing his silver-topped cane, tapped his way back across the yard to the house.

I felt quite chatty as I cleared up and was conscious of myself wittering away to Mason and the other men. They had appeared quite impressed by the whole episode and, whilst saying nothing when their boss had been present, they now responded with the usual rural veterinary quips, such as; 'I'll bring the missus over for yer to have a go on.'

'Don't rush him to get up,' I advised finally, as I

234

prepared to leave. 'But you'd best stay with him until he does.'

It was only when I was well clear of Donhill that I pulled up at a quiet spot, closed my eyes and breathed a gargantuan sigh of relief.

McBean had been called to a calving and was full of apologies at having to leave me to cope alone, but was extremely pleased and relieved that the job had gone satisfactorily.

'The anaesthetic was the biggest hurdle,' he admitted. 'But you got the measure of that all right. I'll buy you a pint tonight.'

I thanked him for his offer, thinking that one would be hardly enough, and spent the rest of the afternoon going about the calls with a permanent grin on my face.

*   *   *

First in for evening surgery were Billy Bent and Peter.

''E's still got the lump,' he said forlornly. 'And he won't eat anything, 'e ain't no better at all.'

Peter was sitting in his usual position on the perch, right next to the wire — a picture of absolute dejection.

'If the lump don't go away, what can you do?' asked Billy.

I lifted the little bird from its cage; there was no resistance. On examination, it was obvious that the liquid paraffin had been ineffective. There was only one course — surgery. The crop would have to be opened and the contents released.

'Peter is going to need a little operation,' I told the young lad. 'Just a small one to empty the "stomach". Well, it isn't really the stomach, it's the part before it called the crop, all part of his digestive system. But it's the only way.' Billy's eyes widened and his lip began to tremble. 'Now look, Billy,' I comforted, 'you leave Peter with me for tonight and I'll see if I can ease that lump. You come round in the morning.'

'I can't come till this time,' he murmured. 'I got papers in the morning.'

I looked at him, standing there, less than four foot high and hardly big enough to keep a newspaper carrier clear of the floor.

'All right, then,' I said. 'You come back tomorrow night.' And I put Peter back inside his cage.

Billy stretched up and passed his hand through the open door to stroke the frail bird's dulled feathers.

'I'll be back for you tomorrow, Pete,' he said, gently. 'Now don' you worry.'

I left Peter until I had cleared the rest of the clients. It wasn't going to be a big job — a whiff of ether, a small nick to remove the debris and a fine stitch would be all that was required. I remembered the miners in Abergranog doing it on their pigeons without much fuss, and they always seemed to make a good recovery.

I checked the procedure in a reference book. There wasn't much on birds, except to say that they were very sensitive and easily shocked. But, as with Warrior, risks had to be taken and my confidence in my abilities as a surgeon had risen considerably since the morning's achievement.

I got a bell jar from the dispensary and a swab of cotton wool. Then the instruments, a scalpel, forceps and fine needle and suture — it seemed quite odd that, although smaller, the needs for both bull and budgerigar were nearly the same.

Carefully I removed Peter from the cage and placed him under the jar. Then quickly I moistened the cotton wool with ether and slipped it in after him.

The bird made no move to panic or flutter about. He just stood there, head gently nodding. Then I noticed the third eyelid becoming more prominent — the ether was obviously having its effect. Peter opened his beak as if to yawn, then he shuddered and fell over on his side.

236

I left him for a few seconds to ensure he was fully anaesthetised, then lifted the jar, withdrew the tiny feathered
scrap and laid it on the table.

He was indeed, very still — there was no movement of
breast feathers or any part of the chest. I moved him gently
with my finger, and as I did so he began to extend his legs,
then his tiny claws clenched and relaxed again — and I
knew that Peter was dead.

Unpredictable death is a terrible thing, an almost unreali-
stic state of affairs, even when it's only a budgerigar.

It's the awful finality and the realisation that things can
never be the same again. Something that everyone, but
vets in particular, must get used to — but at that moment, I
just wasn't used to it. 'Shock' covers it all — and I was
shocked.

Miss Billings was understanding and told me it was not
my fault, which I had already tried to tell myself. In fact, it
was not the budgie for which I was upset — it was for Billy.
Billy, whose parting words, 'I'll be back for you tomorrow.
Now don' you worry,' still rang in my ears.

It was ironic that after all my worry about Warrior and
the consequent success of the morning, instead of finishing work in a state of elation, I drove back to the digs
depressed over the death of a budgerigar.

Meeting Diana that evening cheered me up considerably, and probably I bored her by talking about people and
pets, but she didn't complain. I tried to keep telling myself
that it was just one of those things and I shouldn't get so
involved, but despite all the reasoning, I still wasn't
looking forward to breaking the news to Billy the following
evening.

Warrior looked magnificent when I visited Donhill next
morning.

'Never worried him one bit,' said Mason. 'Give him
some sweet hay last night an' he cleared the lot. Bit tender
behind, but nothing like as lame as he used to be. The boss

ain't half pleased and you're to go to the house when you've finished.'

I gave Warrior another large dose of penicillin and, after satisfying myself that the bandages were still good, I went for my audience with Paxton.

I was ushered into his presence in a grand book-lined study by the greyhaired lady, who didn't introduce herself, but who I assumed was the housekeeper.

The atmosphere reminded me of a film I had recently seen about the President of the United States, for the old man was seated behind a vast oak desk on which were but four objects: a large open book (probably a diary), a pen and holder on a small marble plinth, a photograph in an ornate frame and a silver box. The rest of the room was heavily curtained and a glass-doored showcase crammed with silver cups and trophies stretched the length of the far wall. Every other available wall space was hung with photographs of Hereford cattle, while over an Adam fireplace was an oil painting, unmistakably of Warrior.

'Sit down, Lasgarn,' he said. 'You've seen him, then?'

'Yes,' I replied, 'and he's doing very well.'

He leaned across the desk, opened the silver box and offered me a cigarette. I shook my head and he snapped the lid shut.

'I'm very pleased with you, that was a good piece of work,' he continued, still fixing me with his usual steely glare. There was a silence as if he was waiting for a response. 'Well!' he barked impatiently. 'You can at least smile. I don't usually hand out compliments!'

'Thank you,' I said.

'What's the matter with you, man?' Paxton shouted. 'You look as if you've lost a pound and found sixpence!'

The analogy was so much the opposite that I had to smile. 'No, Mr Paxton,' I replied, 'it's the other way about.'

'What the hell do you mean by that?' he roared.

So I told him all about Billy Bent and his budgerigar.

According to form, he should have leapt up from the desk and berated me for wasting his time, but he didn't, and instead listened intently to everything that I said.

When I had finished, he rubbed his chin rather roughly with his stubby fingers, then shook his head and the faintest of faint smiles ventured from the corner of his mouth.

'Come with me, Lasgarn,' he said, rising from his chair. 'Come with me.'

I followed him through the French windows and along a paved pathway to a door that led into a walled garden. Like everything else at Donhill, the vegetation was flourishing — raspberry canes laden, strawberries in abundance, lettuces, onions, peas and beans, all of the highest quality. Eventually we came to a long, low building where Paxton halted and, taking a key from his waistcoat pocket, unlocked the door.

'Go on in!' he ordered, motioning with his cane. 'See what you think of that!'

He stood back and I walked up the stone steps and into an aviary, the most exotic I could ever have imagined. My entry precipitated an explosion of noise, colour and activity, kaleidoscopic in the extreme. Large airy cages of glossy parakeets, twittering finches, apple-green love-birds, bronze-winged mannikins, sulphur-crested cockatoos and budgerigars by the hundred.

I could do nothing but stand and absorb the fusion of sights and sounds that enveloped my whole person. As if replacing a cork in a bottle, when Paxton closed the door behind him, the cacophony gradually subsided until it was reduced to a melodic harmony and the birds settled on their perches or sank inside their nesting boxes again.

'How about that, then?' asked Paxton proudly.

'Magnificent,' I admitted. 'Absolutely magnificent.'

He leaned against the side of an enclosure which housed at least one hundred Java sparrows, each one immaculate in neat grey plumage, black head and white cheek patches. They fluttered up nervously, rearranging their positions several times until, finally, they calmed and sat, looking down their bulbous, rose-coloured beaks at Paxton and myself.

'I rarely bring anyone in here,' he said. 'This is my place, a place to remind me ...' He straightened up, moving from the support of the enclosure, then leaned forward, both hands on his cane. 'You think I'm an arrogant bastard, don't you?'

I made no comment.

'Go on! Go on! Admit it!'

I nodded.

'Of course you do! Of course you do!' he hissed. 'And you're right, I am!' Paxton straightened up as if proud of the fact, and the Java sparrows twittered nervously and rearranged themselves once again. 'And, Lasgarn, I'll tell you why. I'll tell you why.'

It brought back memories of the Ancient Mariner from my schooldays, for the tale I could not choose but hear.

'When I was a lad,' began Paxton, 'up North and many moons ago, we lived on a large estate.' His upper lip curled malevolently — it was obviously not a happy memory.

'My father worked on the land and my mother was in service — and they were treated like dirt!' Paxton all but spat upon the ground. 'My father died at thirty — worked to death. And my mother — they took advantage of her, too ...' From his eyes, I detected there was more to that than was said. 'I had a pet jackdaw, Barley I called him, because I found him on the edge of a barley field one Summer. His wing was broken and he could only just flitter a few feet from the ground. But I took him home and cared for him, fed him and made a pen in the garden of our cottage. That bird was my whole life.' The old man shook his head and looked up at the roof; he was upset, there was no doubt about it. 'Barley would ride on my shoulder, and if he ever left it, no more than three or four yards he would go, then back he'd come with just enough wing beat to get onto my shoulder again. Well, one day I was walking through the wood to wait for Mother coming home from the Court, when His Lordship's two sons came by. They had three dogs with them, a Springer and two Labradors, one black and one yellow, and when they saw me, the dogs came at me as if I was a hare. I stood my ground, but Barley panicked and fluttered up into a beech tree and wouldn't come down. I called and coaxed, but he wouldn't budge.

'We'll get him down for you,' they said and ran off. 'I thought they were going to get a ladder.' Paxton looked up at the roof again and then closed his hand over his face. 'But when they came back, they had a gun. And the bastards shot Barley right out of the tree.'

For a few moments, he stood, incensed by the memory of the tragedy so indelibly imprinted upon his mind. Then he took a deep breath and continued.

'I was eight at the time, the same age as your Billy Bent. But that experience changed my whole personality. I'd been a quiet, even shy boy before, but after that, I swore I'd get even. And, by God, I did!'

I was eager to ask how, but there was no need, for Paxton was oblivious of my presence, he was re-living his past with all the aggression and venom which life had inflicted upon him.

'I worked, I sweated, I slaved. I bought and sold scrap. Then the War came. The Great War — that was a misnomer, if ever there was one. I saw men killed and killed men myself. I took orders, then I became a sergeant and I gave orders. I was in the thick of it. And I saw officers at the back and soldiers at the front. They even gave me a medal.

'When I came out, Lasgarn, I got back into business and I trod on people and hurt people and barged my way through life. I bought property, then a factory and another factory, went into engineering, until by the time I was fifty I had made a fortune.

'Then the estate where I was born came up for sale, but it was so run-down they couldn't get a bid. And they came and asked me if I was interested. What d'you think of that, Lasgarn? They came and asked the servant's son. And what did I do?' He looked above and beyond me, searching for the golden filmstrip sunset, like the Brigadier on my deferment board. 'I laughed in their bloody faces, Lasgarn, that's what I did. Laughed in their bloody faces!'

Suddenly, as if the emotion had sapped all his energy, he leaned back rather heavily against the sparrow enclosure and I moved forward, thinking he was about to collapse, but he waved his hand to show he was all right.

'So, I sold up and moved down here,' he continued. 'And I decided to have the best — the best land, the best crops, the best livestock — and the finest collection of birds that money could buy.' He waved his cane about expansively. 'And all, Lasgarn, all, you might say, because of a dead jackdaw.'

He was quiet for a while and I was uncertain how to respond. Certainly he wouldn't thank me for any commiseration. Then he smiled briefly and wistfully: 'But I never had any time for anything else. Time to get married, time to raise a family. Oh, I've got some grand nieces that come down from time to time, but they don't come so much now. I'm a successful but miserable old man, Lasgarn, and I don't know why I've told you all this.'

I raised my eyebrows, but made no comment, for indeed, I too was at a loss to know why he had revealed his background to me.

'Billy Bent,' he said, as if that was the answer. 'You bring him out here to see my birds and he shall have the smartest pair of budgerigars in the county to go home with.'

Before I could even thank him, he was motioning for me to leave, and he followed, locking the aviary behind him. We came to another door leading back to the farm. 'What I've told you goes no further, d'you understand,' he grunted, showing me through. 'Don't think I'm asking for sympathy, I'm not! And don't think I'll make life any easier for you, because I won't! I'll ride you as hard as anybody!' I looked back at him as he started to close the door behind me; he was grinning. 'But I know you can take it,' he added. 'Bring that young Billy out on Saturday — and bring that young lady of yours, too. I know she'd like to see my birds.'

With that, he slammed the door, leaving me standing alone on the yard.

*   *   *

Billy didn't cry when I told him that Peter had died — in fact, it might have been easier for me if he had. He just kept searching my face with his sad little eyes as if I had spoken in a foreign language that he didn't understand. I explained that Peter was very weak and the operation was really the only hope, but he didn't respond. Even when I told him of Mr Paxton's offer, he just shrugged his shoulders and said he would have to ask his Gran.

As I had only two further clients, I suggested that, if he waited, I would take him back home in my car and we could then ask his grandmother. That seemed to cheer him up more than anything.

'Can we take Peter home, too?' he asked.

'You're going to bury him?'

He nodded. 'Of course you can,' I said. 'We'll do it together.'

When we arrived, Billy's Gran was sweeping the steps of the little terraced house behind the railway station. I explained about Peter and the proposed visit to Donhill and she was happy about the idea.

'Don't get much attention with his Dad gone and his Mam in hospital,' she admitted.

'How is his mother?' I enquired.

The old lady shook her head, indicating a hopeless situation. 'Matter of months,' she said forlornly. 'But it'll be a blessing. Anyway, a trip in the country will do Billy the world of good. Thank you very much. I'll have him ready at two.'

There was only a postage stamp garden, but Billy chose a spot in the corner of a straggling flower bed and we buried Peter in a cardboard bandage box that I had in the car. Billy put a small ring of stones around the patch.

And so, after laying Peter to rest and promising to call at two o'clock on Saturday, I went back to the digs.

Saturday was hot and dry. The ground lay parched and hard, for there had been little rain for five weeks, but the corn was turning fast and the countryside looked well as we drove out to Donhill. Diana and I had collected Billy at two, looking as if he had been through a laundry and smelling of carbolic.

Paxton acted like a benevolent uncle, a role of which I would never have thought him capable.

The greyhaired lady served tea on the lawn with sandwiches, cakes, strawberries and cream, and Billy ate as if it was his last day on earth. The old man was charm itself to Diana, calling her 'my dear', and guiding her gently by the elbow wherever he took her.

We saw Warrior and the rest of the Hereford cattle, the thoroughbred Arabs, the flock of pedigree Suffolks, the rose gardens, the lake and, finally, the aviary.

Billy looked quite frightened when he first entered, unable to comprehend the sudden intensity of noise and colour. But once he acclimatised, the little lad couldn't stop asking questions, and Paxton answered every one with an equal enthusiasm.

Finally, the old man produced a pair of budgerigars, one green and the other blue, just like Peter, for Billy to take home. And, not only did he provide the birds, but a brand new, brightwired cage with all the equipment as well. Without any prompting, Billy thanked him, and I suspected that both man and boy had tears in their eyes. I know Diana had.

Paxton had said very little to me all afternoon, concentrating entirely on Diana and the boy. It was only when we were leaving that he took much notice of me at all. Billy had run on ahead and climbed the paddock rails to take a last look at the Herefords; then, giving them a wave, he ran back towards us.

'Well, Billy,' said Paxton, 'have you enjoyed yourself?'

'Yes, please. Thank you very much,' Billy replied.

'I suppose that one day, you'd like to be a farmer like me, with all these cows?'

Billy looked back at the grazing herd, then around at the buildings and, finally, towards the great house, as if weighing up the prospects. Then he took hold of Diana's hand and said: 'No, thank you. I'd rather be like Mr Lasgarn.'

Paxton tapped his cane, but once, then turned to face me.

'Lasgarn,' he said, nodding his head gently as if, after much deliberation, he had finally come to a conclusion. 'Lasgarn, I've said this before and I'll say it again: you're a very fortunate fellow.'

And with that, I had to agree.

Ten

Exactly a fortnight later, to the very day, I took Diana to the Shepwall Valley and the Black Mountain. I had taken her for a very special reason, for that morning something had happened that presented yet another crossroads in my life.

I had received a letter from the War Department.

The afternoon was blisteringly hot and there was still no rain. The sky was silver-blue and riding high, with but the merest flecks of cloud to tint it, while beneath, a heat haze shimmered all around. We left the car on the south side and together climbed to a ridge they call the Cat's Back. Diana walked ahead, for the path was narrow, being used mostly by surefooted sheep and wild mountain ponies.

The soft breeze, so welcome after the still, hot air of the valley below, streamed through her fair hair, teasingly pressing the folds of her thin summer dress against the contours of her body. Purposely I held back to watch her — a beautiful girl on a mountain.

Below and all around lay Herefordshire, the natural patchwork now set with yellow, bronze and gold as oats and wheat and long-bearded barley wavered in the sun. I could see Pontavon, far below, where Mrs Williams and her children lived, and farther up, the track to Howell Powell's disappearing behind a hill.

Ledingford lay partly hidden, twelve miles or more to the east, the lofty spire of St Mark's signalling its presence. The river, lazy now and low, with lank green weed and gravel islands in its course, lingered in the parklands where Granstone's towers peeped above the trees. Far in the distance was the rise where Donhill stood. And, standing with my back to Wales, I took in all the peace of the English countryside.

How much I'd come to know and love the county, the people, the livestock and the fulness of their existence. In the early months, I had been like the corn, fresh and green, yet now, after only three short seasons, I felt far more mature — even confident.

Diana had halted and, turning, blew some errant strands of hair from her face.

'Isn't it wonderful,' she said dreamily. 'Don't you wish this could last forever?'

It was then that I brought out the buff envelope.

'I had this, this morning,' I said. 'From the War Department.'

'Oh, Hugh!' she gasped. 'No!'

I opened it and, taking out the letter, read it to her:

I have to inform you that, in view of the reduction of the National Service Commitment, you are exempt from recruitment as from September.

She took a few seconds to take it in, then threw her arms around me.

'Oh! Hugh! How marvellous!' she cried happily. Then I felt her body tense and she drew back. 'Does that mean you'll stay?'

Her face was alight with anticipation, her eyes wide and expectant, lips barely apart.

'On one condition,' I said.

'What's that?' she asked breathlessly.

'That you'll marry me.'

The soft breeze blew, the sun beat down — Diana said 'Yes'.

And that old Black Mountain was the very first to know.

Fontana Paperbacks: Non-fiction

Fontana is a leading paperback publisher of non-fiction. Below are some recent titles.

- [ ] THE LIVING PLANET David Attenborough £8.95
- [ ] SCOTLAND'S STORY Tom Steel £4.95
- [ ] HOW TO SHOOT AN AMATEUR NATURALIST Gerald Durrell £2.25
- [ ] THE ENGLISHWOMAN'S HOUSE
      Alvilde Lees-Milne and Derry Moore £7.95
- [ ] BRINGING UP CHILDREN ON YOUR OWN Liz McNeill Taylor £2.50
- [ ] WITNESS TO WAR Charles Clements £2.95
- [ ] IT AIN'T NECESSARILY SO Larry Adler £2.95
- [ ] BACK TO BASICS Mike Nathenson £2.95
- [ ] POPPY PARADE Arthur Marshall (ed.) £2.50
- [ ] LEITH'S COOKBOOK
      Prudence Leith and Caroline Waldegrave £5.95
- [ ] HELP YOUR CHILD WITH MATHS Alan T. Graham £2.95
- [ ] TEACH YOUR CHILD TO READ Peter Young and Colin Tyre £2.95
- [ ] BEDSIDE SEX Richard Huggett £2.95
- [ ] GLEN BAXTER, HIS LIFE Glen Baxter £4.95
- [ ] LIFE'S RICH PAGEANT Arthur Marshall £2.50
- [ ] H FOR 'ENRY Henry Cooper £3.50
- [ ] THE SUPERWOMAN SYNDROME Marjorie Hansen Shaevitz £2.50
- [ ] THE HOUSE OF MITFORD Jonathan and Catherine Guinness £5.95
- [ ] ARLOTT ON CRICKET David Rayvern Allen (ed.) £3.50
- [ ] THE QUALITY OF MERCY William Shawcross £3.95
- [ ] AGATHA CHRISTIE Janet Morgan £3.50

You can buy Fontana paperbacks at your local bookshop or newsagent. Or you can order them from Fontana Paperbacks, Cash Sales Department, Box 29, Douglas, Isle of Man. Please send a cheque, postal or money order (not currency) worth the purchase price plus 15p per book for postage (maximum postage required is £3).

NAME (Block letters) _____

ADDRESS _____

_____

_____